The Keto Diet: Your Empowering Guide to the Advantages of a High-Fat, Low-Carb Diet.

Ketogenic Cookbook Recipes and Understanding for Rapid Weight loss.

Dr. Michelle Danville

Disclaimer:

© 2017 – TWK - Publishing. All Rights Reserved.

No part of this publication may be reproduced, stored or transmitted in any form or by any means – electronic, mechanical, scanning, photocopying, recording or otherwise, without prior written permission from the author.

This publication is provided for informational and educational purposes only and cannot be used as a substitute for expert medical advice. The information contained herein does not take into account an individual reader's health or medical history.

Hence, it's important to consult with a health care professional before starting any regimen mentioned herein. Though all possible efforts have been made in the preparation of this eBook, the author makes no warranties as to the accuracy or completeness of its contents.

The readers understand that they can follow the information, guidelines and ideas mentioned in this eBook at their own risk. All trademarks mentioned are the property of their respective owners.

Table of Contents

Chapter 1 The Ketogenic Diet: Where it all began 4
   Rediscovery in the modern world 5
   The Science behind the Ketogenic Diet 7
      Getting into Ketosis 11
   How it can help you lose weight and gain energy 12
Chapter 2 Different Cooking Methods 14
   Slow Cooking 15
   Whole Raw Foods 18
   Paleo-Style Ketosis 20
   Blanching 21
   Baking 22
   Roasting 24
   Broiling 24
   Grilling 25
   Sautéing 26
   Pan-Frying 27
   Simmering 27
   Poaching 27
   Steaming 28
   Braising 28
Chapter 3 The Ketogenic Diet as Preventive Medicine 29
   Diabetes 29

Heart Disease Risk Factors 32

Epilepsy 33

Alzheimer's Disease 33

Cancer 34

An important reminder 35

Chapter 4   Whole Food Breakfast Ketogenic Recipes 36

Ketogenic Coffee 36

   Ingredients 36

   Instructions 37

Blueberry Banana Smoothie 37

   Ingredients 37

   Instructions 38

Cauliflower Waffles 38

   Ingredients 38

   Instructions: 39

Keto Pancakes 39

   Ingredients 39

   Instructions: 40

Zucchini Bread 41

   Ingredients 41

   Instructions 42

Ham and Egg Casserole 43

   Ingredients 43

   Instructions 43

No Carb Bagels 44
    Ingredients 44
    Instructions 45
Bacon Breakfast Bagels 46
    Ingredients 46
    Instructions: 46
Classic Bacon and Eggs 47
    Ingredients 47
    Instructions 47
The Keto Breakfast Wrap 48
    Ingredients 48
    Instructions 49
Pumpkin Bread Loaf 50
    Ingredients 50
    Instructions 51
Keto French Toast 52
    Ingredients 52
    Instructions 52
Spinach Scrambled Eggs with Cheddar 53
    Ingredients 53
    Instructions 53
Spinach and Onion Omelette 54
    Ingredients 54
    Instructions 54

Sausage "Egg Muffins" 55
    Ingredients 56
    Instructions 56

Keto No Oat Porridge 58
    Ingredients 58
    Instructions 58

High Fiber Cereal with Cacao Nibs 58
    Ingredients 59
    Instructions 59

Hemp Seed Porridge 61
    Ingredients 61
    Instructions 62

Mocha Chia Pudding 62
    Ingredients 63
    Instructions 63

Egg Porridge 64
    Ingredients 64
    Instructions 64

Cream Cheese Pancakes 65
    Ingredients 65
    Instructions 65

Pumpkin Pancakes 66
    Ingredients 66
    Instructions 67

Carb Free Granola 68
    Ingredients 68
    Instructions 69
White Cheddar and Sausage Biscuits 69
    Ingredients 69
    Instructions 70
Breakfast Frittata with Fried Avocado and Black Olives 71
    Ingredients 71
    Instructions 72
Zucchini Breakfast Hash 72
    Ingredients 73
    Instructions 73
Fisherman's Eggs 74
    Ingredients 74
    Instructions 74
Roasted Tomato Shakshuka 75
    Ingredients 75
    Instructions 75
Green Buttered Eggs 76
    Ingredients 77
    Instructions 77
Breakfast Sausage 78
    Ingredients 78
    Instructions 78

Chapter 5 Whole Food Lunch Ketogenic Recipes 80

Simple Olive Oil Dressing 80
- Ingredients 80
- Instructions 80

Keto Ranch Dressing 81
- Ingredients 81
- Instructions 81

Keto Caesar Dressing 82
- Ingredients 82
- Instructions 82

Tzatziki Sauce 83
- Ingredients 83
- Instructions 83

Basil Salad Dressing 84
- Ingredients 84
- Instructions 84

Cilantro Lime Dressing 84
- Ingredients 85
- Instructions 85

Green Keto Dressing 85
- Ingredients 85
- Instructions 86

Bacon Mustard Dressing 86
- Ingredients 86

Instructions 87
Chicken, Bacon, Avocado Caesar Salad 87
    Ingredients 87
    Instructions 88
Cheese Pizza Rolls 88
    Ingredients 88
    Instructions 88
Broccoli Alfredo Fried Pizza 90
    Ingredients 90
    Instructions 90
Mushroom and Walnut Cauliflower Grits 92
    Ingredients 92
    Instructions 92
Cauliflower Crust Pizza 94
    Ingredients: 94
    Instructions: 94
Oven Roasted Caprese Salad 96
    Ingredients 96
    Instructions 96
Italian Cheesy Bread 97
    Ingredients 97
    Instructions 98
Salmon Patties with Fresh Herbs 100
    Ingredients 100

Instructions 101
Sesame Tofu and Eggplant "Noodles" 102
    Ingredients 102
    Instructions 102
Keto Okonomiyaki 104
    Ingredients 104
    Instructions 105
Quick Keto Egg Drop Soup 106
    Ingredients 107
    Instructions 107
Crispy Tofu and Bok-Choy Salad 107
    Ingredients 108
    Instructions 108
Brie and Apple Crepes 109
    Ingredients 109
    Instructions 110
Low-Carb Guacamole 111
    Ingredients 111
    Instructions 112
Chipotle Steak Bowl 112
    Ingredients 113
    Instructions 113
Chicken Salad Stuffed Avocado 114
    Ingredients 114

Instructions 114

Quick Keto Smoothie Bowl 115

    Ingredients 115

    Instructions 115

Feta and Pesto Omelette 116

    Ingredients 116

    Instructions 116

Spiced Pumpkin Soup 117

    Ingredients 117

    Instructions 118

Buffalo Chicken Soup 119

    Ingredients 119

    Instructions 120

Split Pea and Ham Soup 121

    Ingredients 121

    Instructions 122

Keto Grilled Cheese Sandwich 123

    Ingredients 123

    Instructions 123

Chapter 6 Whole Food Dinner Ketogenic Recipes 125

Creamy Garlic Chicken 125

    Ingredients 125

    Instructions 126

Loaded Mashed "Potatoes" 126

- Ingredients 126
- Instructions 127

Keto Salisbury Steak with Mushroom Gravy 128
- Ingredients 128
- Instructions 129

Garlic Butter Brazilian Steak 130
- Ingredients: 130
- Instructions: 131

Garlic Shrimp Noodles 131
- Ingredients 132
- Instructions 132

Blackened Salmon with Avocado Salsa 133
- Ingredients 133
- Instructions 133

Roasted Shrimp and Asparagus in Lemon, Butter, and Garlic 134
- Ingredients 134
- Instructions 135

Cashew Chicken 136
- Ingredients 136
- Instructions 137

Sausage Casserole 138
- Ingredients 138
- Instructions 139

Ricotta Stuffed Salmon Rolls 140
- Ingredients 140
- Instructions 141

Keto Spaghetti ala Carbonara 142
- Ingredients 142
- Instructions 142

One Pot Shrimp Alfredo 144
- Ingredients 144
- Instructions 144

Eggplant Bacon Alfredo 145
- Ingredients 145
- Instructions 146

Roasted Sea Bass with Herbed Cauliflower Salad 147
- Ingredients 147
- Instructions 147

Nacho Steak Skillet 148
- Ingredients 148
- Instructions 149

Savory Italian Baked Egg 151
- Ingredients 151
- Instructions 151

Hasselback Marinara Chicken 152
- Ingredients 152
- Instructions 153

Roasted Herbed Chicken with Brussels Sprouts Side ...154
- Ingredients ...154
- Instructions ...155

Mississippi Roast ...156
- Ingredients ...156
- Instructions ...157

Coconut-Lime Skirt Steak ...157
- Ingredients ...158
- Instructions ...158

Deconstructed Pizza Casserole ...159
- Ingredients ...159
- Instructions ...159

Cabbage Lasagna ...161
- Ingredients ...161
- Instructions ...161

Cheddar-Wrapped Taco Rolls ...163
- Ingredients ...163
- Instructions ...165

Lamb Meatballs with Cauliflower "Rice" Pilaf ...167
- Ingredients ...167
- Instructions ...168

Cheesy Spinach Rolls with Apple Slaw ...169
- Ingredients ...169
- Instructions ...170

Chicken and Bacon Patties 172
    Ingredients 172
    Instructions 172

Keto Quarter Pounder 173
    Ingredients 173
    Instructions 174

Pepperoni and Cheese on Cheese Crust Pizza 175
    Ingredients 176
    Instructions 176

Cheddar Chicken and Broccoli Casserole 177
    Ingredients 178
    Instructions 178

Ultimate Cheeseburger Loaf 179
    Ingredients 179
    Instructions 180

Chapter 7 30 Whole Food Desserts Ketogenic Recipes ... 184
    Coco Butter Fat Bombs 184
    Ingredients 184
    Instructions 184

    Berries and Cream Fat Bombs 185
    Ingredients 185
    Instructions 186

    Choco Peanut Butter Bombs 187
    Ingredients 187

Instructions 187

No-Bake Choco Peanut Butter Fudge 188

    Ingredients 188

    Instructions 189

Chai Spice Mug Cake 189

    Ingredients 189

    Instructions 190

Mug Churro 190

    Ingredients 191

    Instructions 191

PB Choco Chunk in a Mug 192

    Ingredients 192

    Instructions 193

Coco Choco Mocha Mug Cake 193

    Ingredients 193

    Instructions 194

Pecan Butter Ice Cream 194

    Ingredients 195

    Instructions 195

Keto Strawberry Ice Cream 195

    Ingredients 196

    Instructions 196

Classic Vanilla Ice Cream 197

    Ingredients 197

  Instructions 197

 Mocha Pudding Cake 198

  Ingredients 198

  Instructions 199

 Keto Coffee Cake 200

  Ingredients 200

  Instructions 201

Chapter 8 Snack Ketogenic Recipes 203

 Spicy Cheese and Sausage Dip 203

  Ingredients 203

  Instructions 204

 Cheesy Onion Dip 204

  Ingredients 205

  Instructions 205

 Pizza Dip 206

  Ingredients 206

  Instructions 206

 "Bread" Sticks 207

  Ingredients 207

  Instructions 208

 Kale Chips 209

  Ingredients 209

  Instructions 209

 Green Bean Fries 209

- Ingredients 210
- Instructions 210
- Tropical Smoothie 211
  - Ingredients 211
  - Instructions 211
- Spinach and Cucumber Smoothie 212
  - Ingredients 212
  - Instructions 212
- Hearty Red Smoothie 212
  - Ingredients 213
  - Instructions 213
- Green Smoothie 213
  - Ingredients 213
  - Instructions 214
- Conclusion 215

Introduction

With the number of people following a ketogenic diet, it is no surprise why this diet has been gaining attention as of late. Add to the fact that female celebrities like Gwyneth Paltrow, Megan Fox, and Kim Kardashian are known to follow this diet, it is no surprise that a simple Google search for the term "ketogenic diet" would give you thousands of results on guides and recipes. But, before anyone decides to venture into this kind of diet, it's important to first get the facts straight. So, what is the ketogenic diet?

The ketogenic diet is a macronutrient regimen that puts your body in a state wherein it primarily uses fat to meet energy requirements. It achieves this through a natural metabolic process called Ketosis. The ketogenic diet is done by removing most of the sugars and starches in your diet and following a high healthy fat, moderate protein, low carbohydrate diet. But, as you will discover in the first chapter, the concept of inducing ketosis is not as new as you might think.

As for how it can affect one's personal life, I can attest to its positive effects on both body and confidence. I have always had difficulty of losing weight, particularly fat. I do exercise from time to time but I am not one of those girls you would constantly see in gym clothes. And, add my love for food and anything delicious, one could say that I have found it difficult to get my weight down at levels that I could say I would look and feel my best. Of course, when I don't look, and especially feel my best, I don't do that well in social settings, in work, and in dating.

In my attempts to overcome my struggles with weight loss, I came across the ketogenic diet. At first, it sounded too good to be true because it does not require me to meticulously count calories or to sacrifice my desires of having good food. But, as you will find out in the third chapter of this book, I have found out that it has its history in the medical field and has sufficient amount of research in regards to its effects on weight loss. Because of this, I gave my commitment to the diet and I, eventually, achieved the best body that gave me the confidence to do better in every area of my life.

As a result of my efforts, I have discovered recipes that let me pursue my physical goals without sacrificing the taste I have for food. These recipes have aided me, and now I am offering these to you to help you achieve a better body in looks and in health. With these recipes, you're already a step closer to realizing your goals.

Chapter 1
The Ketogenic Diet: Where it all began

As early as 400 B.C., ancient Greek physicians treated their patients from diseases, particularly epilepsy, by designing a diet that goes out of their usual norm. A dissertation entitled "On the Sacred Disease" found in the "Hippocratic Corpus" indicates that epilepsy is believed to be supernatural in origin, but argued that, although physical and rational in approach, a dietary therapy is an effective cure. This point is reiterated by a different dissertation, entitled Epidemics, in the same collection – revealing the case of a man with epilepsy whom was quickly cured through total abstinence from food and drink. The same point was expressed by Greek Royal Physician and anatomist, Erasistrus, and by Aelius Galenus, a Greek physician, philosopher, and surgeon, in their separate works.

Rediscovery in the modern world

In 1911, a study was conducted by French physicians to see if there was any basis to what Greek medical practitioners were saying in the surviving copies of the Hippocratic Corpus. Twenty epilepsy patients of various ages were assigned a vegetarian diet that is low on calories with a periodic cycle of fasting and excretion. Those who were able to follow the eating regimen gained tremendous benefits for their condition.

The study was noticed by other medical practitioners around the globe and started advocating the nutritional regimen for epileptics. One of these doctors was Hugh Conklin, an osteopathic physician from Battle Creek, Michigan, U.S.A. He adopted an approach that had the patient only ingesting water for a period of eighteen to twenty-five days. He was able to treat hundreds of patients with epilepsy and observed a 90% success rate among children and 50% success rate among adults. He explains that this is due to epileptic seizures being caused by a toxin in the intestines.

Practicing neurologists heard of the success from Dr. Conklin's treatments and they started treating their patients in the same way. These neurologists have observed the same improvements from their patients. But, they observed that the benefits only lasted during the duration of the patient's fasting. Eventually, researchers have pinpointed ketosis as the main cause of the therapeutic effect for epileptic seizures.

Prior to 1922, the only known method to achieve ketosis is through fasting. It was thanks to the study by Dr. Stanley Cobb, a neuropathologist at Harvard Medical School, which gave light to how it is achieved. In due course, various metabolic balance studies used the results of this study and his further studies to understand the relationships between the metabolism of carbohydrates, proteins, and fats by our body. Hence, it was discovered that a diet rich in fats and low in carbohydrates can also help put the body in a state of ketosis.

The Science behind the Ketogenic Diet
To understand the science behind this diet, it is important to have a basic understanding of how our bodies get the energy it needs from the food we eat. The food we eat is digested to break it down via mechanical and chemical action into simpler forms that our body can utilize. These simpler forms come in the form of macronutrients and micronutrients. For the purposes of explaining ketosis, we would be focusing on the three macronutrients: carbohydrates, proteins, and fats.

- *Carbohydrates*

The sugars and starches from grains, fruits, and vegetables in our diet are called carbohydrates. Its digestion begins from the very moment we start chewing with our mouth and mixing it with our saliva. It is then further broken down and absorbed by our small intestine for it to be processed into either glucose, sucrose, or fructose by our pancreas.

Out of the simpler forms of carbohydrates, our bodies prefer glucose as it can be easily circulated from our digestive system to the different parts of our body. As for the other two, sucrose still requires to be further broken down into either glucose or fructose, while fructose can only be metabolized by our liver.

- *Proteins*

We get protein from meat, dairy products, eggs, nuts, and beans that we incorporate into our diet. These are broken down by the stomach, absorbed through the small intestines, and processed by the pancreas into amino acids. Amino acids are used to form neurotransmitters, and to create non-essential amino acids and other protein compounds. Any amino acids in excess are distributed throughout our body for the repair of damaged tissues; creation of enzymes and hormones for various chemical reactions and processes; maintenance of the collagen that gives form to bone structure; creation of antibodies for our immune system; and for storage as glucose.

- *Fats*

Fats come from the different oils and fats that we get from our food. These are broken down by our liver and pancreas into simpler and more useful forms known as fatty acids and glycerol. Our body uses fatty acids and glycerol to repair cells, to create new cells and tissues, and to make different chemicals for our bodily functions.

But, aside from the mentioned functions of fat and its simpler forms, fat can also be used as a source of energy. This happens by having the body's different fat cells release stored up triglycerides. These triglycerides are converted by the liver into ketone bodies through a process called Ketogenesis. These ketone bodies serve as an alternative fuel source for cells found in the brain, kidneys, muscles, and intestines. Once they are provided to these cells, enzymes convert ketone bodies into acetyl CoA through a process called Ketolysis. At this state, which is called ketosis, you will have elevated ketone bodies in your bloodstream due to the needs of your cells for energy.

The modern diet is rich in carbohydrates and this caused our bodies to be highly dependent on glucose as an energy source. This dependence made it hard for our body to get into a state of ketosis whenever blood sugar goes down. And, when blood sugar goes down, the body just signals for the brain to kick up the signs for hunger – prompting you to seek sustenance despite having an abundant source of energy in the form of fat. As a result, your body is in a cycle of gaining fat from excess caloric intake, incapable of using body fat as a source of energy.

With the ketogenic diet being high in fats and low in carbohydrates, your body gets to familiarize itself again with metabolizing fats.

This results into fat loss and decreased fat gain due to your body being less demanding for energy needs. Furthermore, once your body gets back into its normal cycle of carbohydrate and fat metabolism, you will have a more manageable appetite due to the appetite suppressing hormones, ghrelin and leptin, that result from ketosis.

Getting into Ketosis

Around 2 to 8 hours after your last dinner, your body enters a state of fasting. This means your body's glucose drops at a lower limit level, which additionally cuts down the presence of insulin in your blood. With the drop of glucose in your blood, a hormone from the liver, called glucagon, is secreted. This results to the release of glucose and fat into the bloodstream.

Soon, the body begins to enter a ketogenic state. Triglycerides are discharged from fat cells and are utilized by your muscles and liver cells as fuel. From the liver's utilization of triglycerides, ketones are shaped and utilized if more vitality is required. As your body's fasted state goes further, more triglycerides are discharged, separated, and utilized for energy.

There are two ways through which ketosis can be achieved. You could either fast or simply substitute the carbohydrates in your diet with healthy fats. Since fasting in the long-term is not a sustainable way to achieve ketosis, the ketogenic diet is the way to go for anyone who wants to take advantage of this fat-burning state.

However, the ketogenic diet goes beyond maintaining the right ratio of carbohydrates, proteins, and fats in your meals. You must eat the right nutrients to be able to healthily achieve ketosis. Doing so otherwise could lead to chronic inflammation, metabolic disorders, and other degenerative diseases.

How it can help you lose weight and gain energy
Our bodies can originally process both glucose and fatty acids as a source of energy. But, since the average modern diet is rich in starch and simple carbohydrates, our bodies

have gotten used to using glucose, the simple and broken down form of carbohydrates, as its primary fuel. With the body used to glucose as a fuel source, it finds it hard to start up ketosis when its blood sugar levels drop. The result is that you experience a state of light-headedness, decreased mental faculty, and a craving for sugary food.

With a ketogenic diet, you are regaining your body's natural capability to use both fatty acids and glucose as fuel. And, when you use up all the glucose and the fatty acids you have gained from your diet, your body will turn to its fat stores. As you maintain this diet, your body will more often turn to your fat for energy to burn. Eventually, you will notice that you're losing weight without losing muscle.

Chapter 2
Different Cooking Methods

With this being a cookbook, it is important to share a bit of knowledge on food preparation methods. Proper ways of cooking food are often not given the same importance as to what to eat or cook in regards to one's health. But, inadequately cooked food could lead to food poisoning which is just as harmful as eating food with unhealthy ingredients. So, in this vein, I have included a brief introduction and provided some tips on the cooking methods that you would use for the recipes in this cookbook.

Slow Cooking

Slow cooking is a method of cooking that simmers dishes that would normally be boiled. This is done with a product known as a slow-cooker or a crockpot, which simmers food at a lower temperature than cooking methods like baking, boiling, and frying. To cook with this method, the recipe must be made specifically or modified for slow cooking. With little evaporation due to its lower temperature, you would have to make sure that you would end up with the appropriate amount of liquid after cooking.

The most sought-after benefit of slow cooking is its softening effect on the connective tissues of meat without toughening the proteins in the muscle. Furthermore, since slow cooking would usually take the whole day, many found it convenient to just put in the ingredients and come back after their day's work to a hot tasty meal.

But, it has its disadvantage of losing vitamins and minerals in vegetables with how heat breaks down these nutrients. Blanching the vegetables that you would put into a slow cooker would render the enzymes that break down important nutrients ineffective. Other than the disadvantage of potential nutrient loss, frequent removal of the lid would make it difficult for the slow cooker to fully cook the meal. So, if you're planning to cook a perpetual stew like pot au feu or olla podrida, it would be best to stick to the stove top.

To get the best tasting slow-cooked dish, follow the following tips:

- If you're adapting a recipe for slow cooking, use a third less of the total liquids in the ingredients. A slow cooker won't boil your dish and because of this, you would have more liquid left after you're done cooking.
- Brown meat to add color to your dish before you put it in the slow cooker. This would add flavor and texture as well.
- Cuts of meat with a lot of connective tissue work the best with a slow cooker.

Avoid using lean cuts of meat like chicken breast and the more expensive cuts of beef. Cooking lean cuts of meat for a long time would give you a rubbery and tough piece of meat.
- Add dairy products at a much later stage of your cooking. Adding milk, cheese, yogurt, or sour cream too soon will cause these to curdle and ruin your meal.
- It's recommended to minimize the use of wine and liquor or just completely remove these ingredients from the recipe. A slow cooker won't reduce the spirit due to its lower cooking temperature and you would end up with a harsh tasting dish. If you browned a meat for slow cooking, you can deglaze the pan you used with wine or liquor and add the resulting liquid to the slow cooker.

IMPORTANT! If you're planning to incorporate raw beans into an ingredient you would use for slow cooking, you have to boil it for at least 30 minutes at 100 degrees C or 212 degrees F before you put it in the crockpot. Raw beans (like kidney beans, broad beans, and fava beans) contain phytohemagglutinin, which is a toxin that can cause nausea, severe and sustained vomiting, and diarrhea. The reason why this is only a concern for slow cooking is due to the lower cooking temperature that can't destroy the toxin unlike boiling or stewing.

Whole Raw Foods

The whole raw food diet is the practice of eating mostly, if not only, foods that are uncooked and unprocessed. The practice is founded on three claims regarding cooked food:

- Heating food at temperatures of 40 to 48 degrees C (104 to 118 degrees F) breaks down enzymes that can aid digestion.

- Raw foods have greater nutrient and antioxidant content than those that have been cooked.
- Cooked food contains harmful substances like trans fatty acids, acrylamide, advanced glycation end products, and polycyclic aromatic hydrocarbons. To be clear, these substances are present only in poorly prepared and lower quality cooked food. The diet mostly consists of raw fruits, vegetables, seeds, nuts, and sprouted grains. Animal products are mostly avoided due to the cooking or processing required before they're fit for consumption. But, some incorporate whole unpasteurized dairy products, raw eggs, raw fresh fish, and meat into their whole raw foods diet. Preparation can be demanding as raw foods require extra effort in washing the food, and in dehydrating and blending ingredients. Due to the risks involved with this diet, it is not recommended for children, pregnant women, seniors, those who

have a weakened immune system, and those with a chronic medical condition.

Paleo-Style Ketosis

The paleo diet only consists of food presumed to be already available to humans during the Paleolithic era. Foods eaten in this diet include grass-fed meat, organic and sustainable fish and seafood, fresh fruits and vegetables, organic eggs, nuts and seeds, and organic oils from olive, flaxseed, walnut, coconut, and avocado. Foods that are prohibited include dairy products, cereal grains, legumes, refined sugar and carbohydrates, potatoes, processed food, salt, and refined oils like vegetable oils and palm oil.

The rationale behind this diet is that we are genetically adapted to this way of eating due to the availability of these foods before agriculture and food processing even began. Proponents further argue that our bodies are still designed for this diet because adaptation would take a long time before we even get fully used to simple carbs and processed food.

As to be expected, following the paleo diet cuts heart disease risk.

A paleo-style ketosis diet still follows paleo's core concepts but requires very little carbohydrate consumption while maintaining high fat intake – to promote ketosis in the body.

Blanching

Blanching is a process wherein fruits or vegetables is immersed in boiling water for a very brief time and then immediately submerged into iced water to stop it from cooking any further. Aside from partially cooking fruits and vegetables, the result of blanching would often be a softened ingredient and a milder taste. Fibrous vegetables like broccoli, collard greens, and green beans would greatly benefit from blanching as you would end up with tender, yet firm, vegetables while shortening the cooking time.

Regardless of what vegetable you would blanch, the process and the required tools remain the same. You would need a large pot, salt, tongs, a colander for straining, and a bowl full of iced water. You would have to boil water in the pot and add at least a fourth cup of salt per gallon of water. Use the tongs to gently drop the vegetables in the boiling pot of water. After thirty to sixty seconds, test the vegetables for doneness. If the vegetables are ready, transfer them into a colander submerged in iced water.

Dry the vegetables and they're ready to either serve or add to your dish. It would take a bit of practice to know when a particular vegetable is ready but, if you do it right, you would end up with something soft and brightly-colored.

Baking
Baking is a cooking method that utilizes sustained dry heat – usually in an oven. Baked goods typically lack structure before they go in the oven and become solid during the cooking process. In this cooking method, temperatures usually reach up to 375 degrees Fahrenheit.

The most important thing to remember when it comes to baking is to accurately follow what's stated in the recipe. There's little to no room for error in the process and deviating a bit from the required amounts could make the end-product inedible or, at the very least, of poor quality.

Also, keep in mind that not all ovens are the same. One oven might have a different heat distribution compared to another. This could create different results with your baked recipes even if you strictly follow a recipe. To counteract this, you have to be familiar with your oven's unique hot spots. You can test for the hot spots of your oven by laying sliced bread on a cookie sheet and baking at 350 degrees Fahrenheit until color starts to develop. The resulting colorization would tell you where the hot spots are based on the position of dark spots on the bread.

Lastly, keep in mind that most ovens do not have accurate temperature gauges. Because of this, it's recommended to place an oven thermometer inside and use it as basis during pre-heating.

Roasting

Similar to baking, roasting is a cooking method that uses prolonged dry heat. The difference is that food items that are typically roasted already have a solid structure before even the cooking process starts. Also, roasting requires at least 400 degrees Fahrenheit to cook the food and to create the caramelized crust that adds flavor and texture to the dish.

To get the best out of roasting using an oven, almost the same tips in baking applies – and yes, it's crucial that you use a thermometer. In addition to these, make sure to avoid overcrowding your pan as this would make it hard for the air to heat up the food on all sides. And, before carving your roasted meat, allowing it to rest at half the total roasting time is key if you want juicy and moist cuts.

Broiling

Broiling is a cooking method that utilizes direct heat above the food. This is quite popular since it produces a crispy outer texture without drying out the inside. It is best used for thin and lean cuts of meat like poultry cutlets, meat chops, and fillets. But, if the cut is too lean, the meat could dry very quickly and result in a bland tasting dish. In this case, using glaze or marinade is advisable to improve flavor.

Remember that broiling will cook a dish faster than other cooking methods. So, if your recipe calls for broiling, make sure that you closely follow the specified cooking time. And, if you're adapting a recipe for broiling, you can cut the cooking time in half and closely monitor for the desired doneness at that point.

Grilling

Like broiling, grilling is a cooking method that utilizes direct heat. But, unlike broiling, grilling involves heat coming from below the food being cooked. Since grilling can cook food quickly, it is best used with tender cuts of meat, fish, or poultry with the appropriate marinade to prevent drying. Vegetables can also be grilled but would only require a short cooking time.

Sautéing

Sautéing is a cooking method that utilizes a very hot cooking surface, usually a pan or griddle, and a bit of fat. With this method, the food can be cooked very quickly and be browned to develop unique aroma and flavors. To sauté, it is important to get the cooking pan very hot before adding the oil and food, respectively. If the oil is adequately hot, you'll get a sizzling sound after adding the other ingredients.

To get the most out of sautéing, avoid overcrowding the pan with too much ingredients. Overcrowding it can make it difficult for the pan to heat up evenly and sufficiently. This would result in boiling and the sizzle would eventually be absent. In addition, while sautéing, you would want to keep the ingredients moving on the pan by flipping or tossing. This would ensure that the ingredients are evenly cooked and browned.

Pan-Frying

Sautéing and pan-frying are both similar in the sense that they use a hot cooking surface and little cooking oil. The difference is that there is no tossing involved and the temperature much lower. Pan-frying is ideal for cooking larger pieces of meat.

Simmering

Simmering is a cooking method that submerges food in liquid at constant temperatures of 180 to 205 degrees Fahrenheit. Gently rising bubbles are the sign that a cooking liquid is at an adequate simmer. This cooking method is best for preparing soups, stocks, or starchy produce like pasta and root crops.

Poaching

Poaching is a cooking method that also submerges food to cook it. Unlike simmering though, poaching uses a lower range of temperatures (140 to 180 degrees Fahrenheit), and would only last for a short time. The sign that the cooking liquid is ready for poaching is the formation of small bubbles at the bottom of the pot. Due to it gentler temperatures, poaching is best used for delicate food items like fish and eggs.

Steaming

With this method, ingredients are not agitated, which prevents nutrient loss due to leaching. Because of the gentler application of heat, steaming is a good cooking method for vegetables and fish.

Braising

Braising is a combination of cooking methods. It starts with searing the meat to give texture and flavor, and then finishes with a long simmer at low temperatures. This cooking method is best for tougher cuts of meat since it can dissolve tough connective tissues. The simmering part of this cooking method can be done on a stovetop or in the oven.

Chapter 3
The Ketogenic Diet as Preventive Medicine

Proponents of the ketogenic diet claim that it can prevent, and in some cases even cure, various diseases. Surely, there are those who merely exaggerate the diet's benefits, and are clearly downplaying its limitations. In this chapter, you will discover the truth be about the diet's potential.

Diabetes

Diabetes is a collection of metabolic diseases that ultimately manifest in the body in the form of constantly elevated blood sugar levels. This elevated blood sugar is either due to insufficient insulin production or to insensitivity to the insulin produced. Those who have insufficient insulin production usually inherit this trait and are considered to suffer from type 1 diabetes. Type 2 diabetics, on the other hand, developed the condition due to unhealthy body weight, lack of exercise, and poor eating habits.

Given that type 2 diabetes is borne out of an individual's choices, one can say that it can be also managed with better choices regarding one's diet and other lifestyle habits. A 2005 study conducted by researchers from Duke University Medical Center has confirmed the importance of one's diet in reducing the gravity of the disease. The researchers studied 28 overweight individuals with type 2 diabetes for 16 weeks; the participants ate only 20 grams of carbohydrates in a day and reduced their diabetes medication. Those who successfully followed the regimen had an average of 16.6% decrease in their Hemoglobin A1C, a marker for blood sugar level, and aside from this, their triglyceride levels dropped by 41.6%.

Still, experts remain wary of the ketogenic diet, mainly in relation to the possibility of increasing susceptibility towards other chronic diseases. In this vein, Manny Noakes conducted a study in 2006, observing 83 non-diabetic individuals with ages averaging at 43 and an average BMI of 33. The test subjects were divided into three groups, each with a different diet despite all having the same total caloric intake. At the end of the study, although all three groups experienced similar improvements in weight and body fat, the group with a diet consisting of 4% carbohydrate, 20% protein, and 61% fat had the greatest improvement in their triacylglycerol levels, HDL cholesterol levels, and fasting and after-meal glucose and insulin concentrations.

Due to these results, it was concluded that a ketogenic diet can be a successful preventive measure for diabetes – provided that cholesterol levels are closely monitored.

Heart Disease Risk Factors

Heart disease has long been studied and most of its causes are known to be lifestyle related. Recent studies reveal that a high carbohydrate diet is among the main contributors to heart disease. It turns out that the high blood sugar from a carbohydrate-rich diet causes inflammation in the cardiovascular tissues (due to protein glycation). Also, this type of diet increases one's LDL cholesterol while decreasing the levels of HDL cholesterol, which results to a dramatic increase in atherosclerosis risk.

Research has found that the ketogenic diet can greatly decrease the mentioned risks, provided that the diet is nutritionally complete and healthy fats are used. A research by Feinman and Volek in 2006 indicates that, even without weight loss, the lipid profiles (HDL and LDL cholesterol balance) of individuals have improved with a low carbohydrate diet. Furthermore, as discussed in the previous section on diabetes, the ketogenic diet has been proven to keep blood sugar and insulin levels at healthier levels and is seen to improve fasting and post-meal levels. With these two effects in tandem, one can easily see the benefits of a ketogenic diet in the prevention and management of heart disease.

Epilepsy

As discussed in the first chapter, the ketogenic diet was originally a treatment used for epileptic seizures, replacing the initial practice of fasting. Studies have shown that the diet was able to reduce, if not prevent, seizures among patients who have not been able to control it through medication. Tests have shown that seizure occurrences have decreased by at least half and that total seizure prevention has a 10 to 15% chance of success. As to be expected, however, shifting to another diet means that such benefits are lost.

Alzheimer's Disease

Alzheimer's disease is an irreversible brain disorder that develops from simple symptoms of dementia to full-blown loss of one's thinking and memory capacity. Tasks that are simple in nature eventually become difficult to perform. Although the cause for such a disease is still being investigated, research has shown that the Alzheimer's is mainly due to the loss of connection between the brain's neurons.

The success of the ketogenic diet on patients with epilepsy has led researchers to wonder if it could have an effect on those with Alzheimer's disease. A study conducted in 2006 by Gasior, Rogawski, and Hartman has revealed that the ketogenic diet could help protect neurons from further damage and death. This suggests that the diet could be used to slow down and, even, reverse Alzheimer's disease, provided that it is caught in its early stages. But, due to the uncontrolled nature of the study and its focus on animal tests, further research is needed to confirm the diet's viability in the disease's prevention or reversal.

Cancer
Although there is support for the diet's potential in managing cancer, there is still

quite a lot of research needed. A pilot study conducted in 2011 by Shmidt, Pfetzer, suggests that the diet may improve the quality of life of patients with cancer in its advanced stages. Furthermore, a study in 2014 by Allen, Bhatia, Anderson, indicates that the ketogenic diet has anti-cancer effects when done in combination with standard radio-chemotherapy.

An important reminder
The ketogenic diet might have proven and potential health benefits but it is always advised to consult with your doctor if you're suffering from any kind of disease. This book is for informational purposes only and does not suggest that the ketogenic diet can heal whatever disease you currently have.

Chapter 4
Whole Food Breakfast Ketogenic Recipes

Ketogenic Coffee
Prep Time: 5 minutes
Calories: 448
Servings: 1

Ingredients
- 2 cups of coffee
- 2 tbsp unsalted butter from grass-fed cow
- 2 tbsp MCT or coconut oil
- 1 tbsp heavy whipping cream
- 1 tsp vanilla extract

Instructions
1. Brew 2 cups of coffee with the method of your choice.
2. Pour the coffee in a container that can hold an immersion blender.
3. Put the vanilla extract, butter, and coconut oil into the coffee.
4. Blend the mixture with an immersion blender.
5. Add the heavy whipping cream and blend it again with the immersion blender while moving it up and down.
6. Blend it for a minute to get a frothy surface.
7. Serve.

Blueberry Banana Smoothie
Prep Time: 12 minutes
Calories: 592
Servings: 3

Ingredients
- 2 cups unsweetened coconut milk
- ¼ cup blueberries
- 3 tbsp golden flaxseed meal
- 2 tbsp MCT oil or Virgin Coconut Oil

- 1 tbsp chia seeds
- 1 ½ tsp banana extract
- ¼ tsp xanthan gum
- 10 drops liquid stevia

Instructions
1. Combine all the ingredients in a blender.
2. Let the mixture rest for at least ten minutes to let the flaxseed meal and the chia seeds soak in the liquid.
3. Blend for 1-2 minutes until the mixture is smoothly combined.
4. Serve.

Cauliflower Waffles

Cooking Time: 10 minutes
Calories: 705
Servings: 1

Ingredients
- 1 ½ cup grated raw cauliflower
- ½ cup mozzarella
- ½ cup cheddar cheese
- ¼ cup parmesan cheese
- 3 large eggs
- 3 tbsp chopped chives

- ½ tsp onion powder
- ½ tsp garlic powder
- ¼ tsp red pepper flakes
- Salt and pepper to taste

Instructions:
1. Cauliflower can be grated by chopping it and using a food processor's grating attachment
2. Add the cheeses and grate with the food processor.
3. Add the eggs and mix all the ingredients together.
4. Place batter into the waffle maker and cook for about 8 to 10 minutes.
5. Repeat accordingly for the remaining waffle batter.

Keto Pancakes
Cooking Time: 10 minutes
Calories: 520
Servings: 2

Ingredients
- 1 cup almond flour
- ½ cup organic golden flaxseed meal

- ¼ cup almond milk, unsweetened
- ¾ cup ricotta
- 3 large eggs
- 1 tsp. baking powder
- ½ tsp. vanilla extract
- ¼ tsp. salt
- ¼ tsp. stevia powder
- ¼ cup in season fruits of choice (fresh blueberries, strawberries, or bananas work best) or chopped nuts

Instructions:

1. Beat the eggs and mix with the unsweetened almond milk, ricotta, and vanilla extract. You can do this in a blender or add the mixture in a blender for the later steps.
2. In a separate bowl, mix well the almond flour, flaxseed meal, baking powder, salt, and stevia powder.
3. While blending the wet mixture, slowly add the dry mixture to the wet mixture in the blender until a batter forms evenly.
4. For your chosen fruit, how much you add per pancake would depend on your

preference. And, slicing them accordingly would make it easier to place on the pancake and cook.
5. Heat the skillet and add butter.
6. Once the butter has melted, pour an appropriate amount for each pancake batter on the skillet. Flip the pancake once the edges start to get lightly browned.
7. Wait for a minute or two and flip it again to check for doneness. If it's lightly browned, you can take off the pancake from the skillet.
8. You can serve it with sugar-free syrup and fresh fruits.

Zucchini Bread
Cooking Time: 1 hour
Calories: 716
Servings: 2

Ingredients
- 2 ½ cups almond flour
- 1 ½ cups erythritol
- 1 cup grated zucchini
- ½ cup chopped walnuts

- ½ cup olive oil
- 3 large eggs
- 1 ½ tsp baking powder
- 1 tsp vanilla extract
- 1 tsp ground cinnamon
- ½ tsp nutmeg
- ½ tsp salt
- ¼ tsp ground ginger

Instructions

1. Preheat the oven at 350 degrees F.
2. Whisk the eggs with the olive oil and vanilla extract.
3. In another bowl, mix the almond flour, erythritol, baking powder, salt, nutmeg, ginger, and cinnamon.
4. Squeeze out the excess water from the zucchini. You can use your clean bare hands, a paper towel, or a cheesecloth.
5. Add the zucchini into the bowl of the egg mixture. Whisk.
6. Using a hand mixer, slowly add the dry ingredient mixture until fully blended.
7. Lightly spray a loaf pan (9x5 size). Neatly put in the resulting zucchini bread mixture.

8. Cover the zucchini bread mixture with the chopped walnuts. With a spatula, lightly press in the walnuts into the zucchini bread batter.
9. Put it in the oven and bake for 60-70 minutes at the preheated temperature. The bread is done when the crust and the walnuts are browned.

Ham and Egg Casserole

Cooking Time: 30 minutes
Calories: 575
Servings: 3

Ingredients

- 12 large eggs
- 1 pound diced ham
- 1 cup ricotta cheese
- 1 ¼ cup chopped spinach
- ¼ cup heavy whipping cream
- ½ small yellow onion, chopped
- ¼ tsp salt
- ½ tbsp. garlic and herb seasoning

Instructions

1. Preheat oven at 350 degrees F.

2. Whisk four of the eggs and mix until smooth with the heavy whipping cream, onion, and ricotta cheese. Set aside.
3. In a separate bowl, whisk the remainder of the eggs and add it to the previous mixture.
4. Mix in the salt and garlic and herb seasoning.
5. Fold in the diced ham and spinach into the mixture.
6. Spray a casserole dish (preferably 9x13 in size) and pour in the mixture.
7. Put it in the oven to cook for at least 30 minutes or until the top looks thoroughly cooked.

No Carb Bagels
Cooking Time: 18 minutes
Calories: 526
Servings: 1

Ingredients
- ¾ cup almond flour
- 1 ½ cup grated mozzarella
- 1 large egg
- 2 tbsp cream cheese

- 1 tbsp melted butter
- 1 tsp xanthan gum
- Sesame seeds

Instructions

1. Preheat oven at 390 degrees F.
2. Mix the almond flour and xanthan gum in a bowl. Add eggs and mix until thoroughly combined.
3. Slowly melt the mozzarella and cream cheese in a pot over low-medium heat.
4. Add the mixture of melted cheese to the almond flour mixture. Knead until you get it to resemble a dough. When the kneading gets too tough, put it in the microwave for 10-20 seconds before proceeding to knead again.
5. Evenly split the dough into three portions and roll each into round logs. To form into shape, you can use a donut pan for each log or make circles for each and join the two ends and place on a baking sheet.
6. Brush melted butter on top of the uncooked bagles and sprinkle sesame seeds.

7. Put the bagels in the oven for at least 18 minutes or until the top becomes golden brown.
8. Once cooked, take it out and let it cool on a wire rack.

Bacon Breakfast Bagels

Prep Time: 3 minutes
Calories: 797
Servings: 1

Ingredients

- 1 No Carb Bagel
- 2 slices grilled bacon (or any other filling of your choice)
- 1/3 cup arugula leaves
- ½ tbsp. pesto
- 1/3 tbsp. cream cheese

Instructions:

1. Cut the bagel in half. You can toast it before or after cutting depending on whether you want the inside toasted or not.
2. Spread cream cheese inside the bagel. Top it off with pesto.

3. Add the arugula leaves and top it with the bacon or your choice of filling.

Classic Bacon and Eggs

Prep Time: 25 minutes
Calories: 826
Servings: 1

Ingredients
- 4 slices of bacon
- 3 large eggs, room temperature
- 1/3 cup heavy whipping cream
- 1 tbsp butter
- Salt and freshly ground pepper to taste

Instructions
1. Preheat the oven at 350 degrees F.
2. Lay the bacon slices on a baking sheet and put them in the oven once it's fully heated.
3. After 10 to 15 minutes, the bacon should be looking crispy and could be taken out of the oven.
4. Let it rest on the baking sheet to let it cook a little bit more.
5. Break the eggs into a bowl, add the cream, and lightly whisk.

6. Heat the pan to medium low.
7. Add the butter once it's adequately heated.
8. Once the butter has melted, immediately add the eggs.
9. Let the egg mixture properly set on the bottom.
10. Gently stir with a spatula to bring up the bottom. Make sure the whole thing stays intact.
11. Once the bottom has set again, stir it again but this time fold the eggs over to make sure all of the egg is cooked.
12. Take it out of the pan. Add salt and pepper.

The Keto Breakfast Wrap
Cooking Time: 3 minutes
Calories: 632
Servings: 1

Ingredients
- 3 large egg whites
- 5 large eggs
- 2 cups spinach leaves
- ½ cup crumbled feta

- 3 whole sundried tomatoes, chopped
- 4 basil leaves, roughly chopped
- 1 tsp sesame oil
- Olive oil
- ½ tsp salt

Instructions
1. Combine the egg whites, whole eggs, salt, and sesame oil in a bowl.
2. Whisk until the mixture gets slightly foamy. This would take at least 30 seconds to a minute of continuous whisking.
3. Spray a skillet or a pan with cooking spray and heat it up to medium heat.
4. Pour half of the egg mixture onto the skillet and reduce the heat to about between low and medium heat.
5. Once there is no raw egg left in the center, the wrap is fully cooked. Remove it from the pan and place it on a cool plate.
6. Prepare the second wrap in the same way.
7. Place the spinach in the skillet and toss it around until the leaves gently wilt.

You can leave it for a minute longer for softer leaves.
8. Divide the crumbled feta, tomatoes, and basil for filling the two wraps.
9. Fill the wrap in the following order: spinach, feta, basil, and a drizzle of olive oil.
10. Roll the wrap and repeat for the second one.
11. Enjoy your Keto Breakfast Wrap

Pumpkin Bread Loaf
Cooking Time: 40 minutes
Calories: 559
Servings: 3

Ingredients
- 1 cup blanched almond flour
- 2 tbsp ground cinnamon
- 2 tsp ground nutmeg
- 1 tsp ground cloves
- 1 tsp ground ginger
- 1 tsp ground allspice
- 3 large eggs
- ½ cup roasted pumpkin
- 2 tbsp coconut oil

- 1 tbsp Greek yogurt
- ½ tsp baking soda
- 20 drops stevia
- ¼ tsp sea salt

Instructions
1. Preheat the oven at 350 degrees F.
2. Mix the almond flour, baking soda, sea salt, and the spices in a medium to large sized bowl.
3. Mix the eggs, roasted pumpkin, coconut oil, Greek yogurt, and stevia in a separate bowl.
4. Stir the second mixture into the first one until you get a smooth batter.
5. Grease two small loaf pans (or one large loaf pan) and pour the batter into the pan/s.
6. Put it in the preheated oven and let it bake for around 40 to 45 minutes. Test for doneness with a toothpick or knife. If the test insert is clean, the loaf is done.
7. Remove from the oven and let it cool on a wire rack.

Keto French Toast

Cooking Time: 20 minutes
Calories: 758
Servings: 1

Ingredients

- 6 pieces of dry pumpkin bread
- ½ cup whole milk
- 3 large eggs
- a splash of vanilla

Instructions

1. Heat a skillet to medium high heat and melt butter on it.
2. Whisk all the wet ingredients together in a bowl.
3. Soak each slice of pumpkin bread in the mixture for 20 seconds. Then, let the excess mixture drip off before putting it on the hot skillet.
4. Pan-fry each side of the slice until you get a golden brown color for each side.
5. Repeat step 4 for each slice.
6. Serve with butter or toasted coconut.

Spinach Scrambled Eggs with Cheddar

Cooking Time: 15 minutes
Calories: 643
Servings: 1

Ingredients
- 4 cups fresh spinach
- 4 large eggs
- ½ cup cheddar cheese
- 1 tbsp olive oil
- 1 tbsp heavy cream
- Pinch of salt and pepper

Instructions
1. Crack the eggs into a bowl
2. Add the heavy cream, salt, and pepper into the bowl.
3. Whisk the mixture
4. Get a large pan and get it up to high heat.
5. Add the olive oil onto the pan.
6. When the oil starts to smoke, put in the spinach and toss it around the pan. Add salt and pepper to taste.
7. Once the spinach reduces, turn down the heat to medium low.

8. Add in the egg mixture into the pan with the spinach.
9. Stir the eggs when it starts to set.
10. Add the cheddar cheese and stir it in to the mix.
11. When the cheese starts to melt, take it off the heat and serve it on a plate.

Spinach and Onion Omelette
Cooking Time: 15 minutes
Calories: 629
Servings: 1

Ingredients
- 2 cups spinach
- 3 large eggs
- ¼ medium onion
- 1 medium spring onion
- 2 tbsp heavy cream
- 2 tbsp butter
- 1 oz goat cheese
- Salt and pepper to taste

Instructions
1. Slice the onion into long strips.

2. Heat the pan in medium low heat and add the butter.
3. Add onion and sauté it in the butter.
4. Add the spinach and remove the contents of the pan once the spinach wilts.
5. Crack the eggs in a bowl. Add salt and pepper.
6. Pour the egg mixture onto the pan and let it cook on medium low heat.
7. Once the bottom and the edges of the egg mixture set, spoon the spinach and onion on half of the omelette.
8. Place crumbled goat cheese over the spinach and onions.
9. Once the top of the omelette sets, fold the omelette and take it off the pan.
10. Serve it on the plate and garnish with spring onions.

Sausage "Egg Muffins"
Cooking Time: 10 minutes
Calories: 793
Servings: 1

Ingredients
- ¼ lb. raw pork breakfast sausage
- 2 large eggs
- ¼ cup water
- 1 tbsp ghee
- 1 ½ tbsp. guacamole
- Salt and freshly ground black pepper to taste

Instructions
1. Grease the insides of two 3 and a half inch biscuit cutters with melted ghee.
2. Fill one cutter with the sausage meat. Press the meat down to form a patty.
3. Heat a skillet to at least over medium heat. Oil the surface with a tablespoon of ghee.
4. When the ghee is fully melted, place the patty on the pan and cook each side for at least 2 to 3 minutes. To keep the perfectly round shape of the patty, keep the mold with the patty and only remove it when it the patty starts to shrink.
5. Transfer patty to a plate after cooking.

6. Get two small bowls and crack an egg into each bowl. Pierce the yolk of each egg with a fork.
7. Heat a skillet to medium-high heat then oil the surface with a tablespoon of ghee.
8. Once the ghee is fully melted, place two greased biscuit cutter on the pan and pour an egg into each one.
9. Season with salt and pepper to taste.
10. Add the water into the skillet (outside the biscuit cutters).
11. Lower the heat to low and cover the skillet.
12. The egg would take at least 3 minutes before it gets cooked.
13. Line a plate with paper towel and transfer the eggs onto it. Sliding a spatula under the biscuit cutter and egg can make it an easier process.
14. Assemble the Sausage "Egg Muffin". Sandwich the sausage patty and guacamole between the egg muffins.
15. Serve.

Keto No Oat Porridge

Cooking Time: 15 minutes
Calories: 341
Servings: 1

Ingredients

- 2 tbsp Chia Seeds
- 2 tbsp ground flax meal
- ½ cup almond milk
- Stevia to taste

Instructions

1. Combine the ingredients into a pot and put on the stove over medium heat.
2. Stir the mixture frequently until it congeals.
3. Remove from heat and add your choice of toppings.
4. Serve.

High Fiber Cereal with Cacao Nibs

Cooking Time: 45 minutes
Calories: 508
Servings: 2

Ingredients
- 1 cup water
- ½ cup chia seeds
- 4 tbsp hemp hearts
- 2 tbsp coconut oil, melted
- 2 tbsp raw cacao nibs
- 1 tbsp Swerve
- 1 tbsp vanilla extract
- 1 tbsp fine Psyllium powder

Instructions
1. Preheat oven to 285 degrees
2. Combine chia seeds and water in a bowl. Stir well and let it soak for around 5 minutes.
3. Add hemp hearts, coconut oil, Swerve, vanilla extract, and Psyllium powder into the bowl. If you want the cacao nibs to break into smaller pieces, you can add them at this point as well.
4. Mix all the ingredients with a wooden spoon or an electric mixer. Stop when the ingredients are smoothly incorporated into the mixture.
5. If you have not yet added the cacao nibs, add them to the mixture.

6. At this point, you should have a dough with a malleable consistency.
7. Form the dough into a cylindrical shape with your hands and place them on the shiny side of a parchment paper.
8. Flatten the dough on top of the parchment paper with your hands.
9. Cover the dough with another parchment paper, shiny side should touch the dough. With a rolling pin, roll it over until you get to at least ¼ inch thickness.
10. Peel off the top parchment paper and lay on the dough on a baking sheet.
11. Put it on the oven for 15 minutes or until it gets to almost dry.
12. Remove from the oven to flip it to the other side and gently peel off the other parchment paper.
13. Return it to the oven for another 15 minutes or until the top gets almost dry.
14. Remove from the oven and gently peel off the remaining parchment paper.

15. Put it back in the oven and back for another 15 minutes or until it is dry. This could take up to 25 minutes depending on your oven.
16. Remove from the oven and let it cool.
17. Once it's cool enough, cut it into squares with an inch on each side.
18. You can store this in an airtight container up to a maximum of 3 days.

Hemp Seed Porridge

Cooking Time: 45 minutes
Calories: 430
Servings: 1

Ingredients

- 1 cup whole milk
- ½ cup hemp seeds (also known as hemp hearts)
- ¼ cup almond flour (or crushed almonds)
- 2 tbsp ground flax meal
- 1 tbsp chia seeds
- ¾ tsp vanilla extract
- ½ tsp ground cinnamon

- 5 drops stevia

Instructions
1. Add all the ingredients except the almond flour into a small saucepan.
2. Stir the contents of saucepan until it forms a well-combined mixture.
3. Heat the saucepan over medium heat.
4. Once it begins to boil lightly, stir the contents once then let it stay on the heat for 1 to 2 minutes.
5. Remove the saucepan from the heat and stir in the almond flour or crushed almonds.
6. Transfer the porridge into a bowl and top with your choice of toppings. Recommended toppings are chopped Brazil nuts and/or a tablespoon of hemp seeds/hearts.

Mocha Chia Pudding
Cooking Time: 15 minutes
Calories: 708
Servings: 1

Ingredients
- 1/3 cup undiluted coconut cream
- 1/3 cup dry chia seeds
- 2 tbsp. ground coffee beans of your choice
- 2 tbsp. cacao nibs
- 1 tbsp. vanilla extract
- 1 tbsp. Swerve

Instructions
1. In a small saucepan, simmer the ground coffee beans with 2 cups of water for at least 15 minutes or until it reduces into about a cup of brewed coffee.
2. Let the resulting brewed coffee rest and slowly strain it and pour in a bowl.
3. Mix in the coconut cream, Swerve and vanilla extract.
4. Stir the mixture well.
5. Blend chia seeds and cacao nibs into the mixture.
6. Place in serving containers.
7. Chill for at least 30 minutes.
8. Serve. Can be topped with additional cacao nibs.

Egg Porridge

Cooking Time: 10 minutes
Calories: 450
Servings: 1

Ingredients

- 2 large eggs
- 1/3 cup heavy cream
- 2 tbsp. butter from grass-fed cow
- Ground cinnamon to taste
- Stevia or organic sweetener to taste

Instructions

1. Crack the eggs into small bowl and add the cream and your choice of sweetener into it.
2. Give the mixture a little whisk.
3. In a medium saucepan, melt the butter over medium-high heat. Do not let it turn brown.
4. Once the butter has melted, add the egg mixture and mix it thoroughly until it thickens and starts to curdle. Tiny grain-like pieces is the sign that it is starting to curdle.

5. At this point, immediately take it off the heat and transfer to a serving bowl to stop the cooking process.
6. Top the porridge with cinnamon.
7. Serve.

Cream Cheese Pancakes

Cooking Time: 10 minutes
Calories: 428
Servings: 1

Ingredients
- 2 eggs
- 2 oz. cream cheese
- 1 tsp Swerve
- ½ ground cinnamon

Instructions
1. Blend all the ingredients in a blender until smooth.
2. Rest for 2 minutes to let the bubbles settle
3. Heat a pan to medium heat and grease it with butter.

4. Pour ¼ of the batter. Cook it for two minutes then flip it to the other side to cook for a minute.
5. Repeat the last step for the remainder of the batter.
6. Serve with fresh berries.

Pumpkin Pancakes

Cooking Time: 10 minutes
Calories: 576
Servings: 3

Ingredients
- 3 large eggs
- 1 cup coconut cream
- ½ pumpkin puree
- 2 oz freshly ground flaxseed
- 2 oz ground hazelnut
- 1 oz egg white protein
- 1 tsp baking powder
- 1 tbsp. chai masala powder
- 1 tbsp Swerve
- 1 tsp vanilla extract
- 4 drops Stevia

Instructions
1. In a bowl, crack the eggs and mix with coconut cream, pumpkin puree, egg white protein, and vanilla extract. Whisk contents until you get a frothy mixture. This would take around 30 seconds.
2. In another bowl, combine ground flaxseed, ground hazelnut, chai masala powder, baking powder, salt, Stevia, and Swerve. Mix well.
3. Whisk the wet mixture and slowly incorporate the dry mixture into it.
4. The batter is ready when it is a semi-think but pourable mixture. Add ¼ cup of water if it is too dry.
5. Heat a non-stick pan at medium heat and melt a tsp of coconut oil on it.
6. Once melted, adjust the heat to low.
7. Pour one ladle of the batter and cover the pan with a lid. Cook each side for 2 to 3 minutes.
8. Repeat the previous step for the remaining batter.

9. Once done, immediately sprinkle with chai masala powder and garnish with whole hazelnuts.
10. Top with coconut cream and serve.

Carb Free Granola

Cooking Time: 20 minutes
Calories: 687
Servings: 8

Ingredients
- 2 cups chopped pecans
- 1 ¾ cup egg white protein
- 1 ¼ cup grass-fed butter or coconut oil, melted
- 1 cup sunflower seeds
- ½ cup slivered almonds
- ½ cup sesame seeds
- ½ cup chopped walnuts
- ½ cup erythritol
- 1 tsp stevia glycerite
- 1 tsp cinnamon
- ½ tsp salt

Instructions
1. Preheat the oven at 300 degrees F.
2. In a large bowl, combine the seeds, nuts, egg white protein, erythritol, cinnamon, stevia, and salt.
3. Pour the butter or coconut oil on the mixture.
4. Thoroughly mix the ingredients together.
5. Lay the mixture onto a baking sheet with edges.
6. Put in the oven to bake for at least 20 minutes or until golden brown.
7. Remove from the oven and let it cool.
8. Break the granola into pieces and store in an airtight container to preserve.

White Cheddar and Sausage Biscuits
Cooking Time: 25 minutes
Calories: 544
Servings: 2

Ingredients
- 1 ½ cup almond flour
- 1 cup white cheddar cheese (sharp or regular)

- ¼ cup heavy cream
- ¼ cup water
- 6 oz ground sausage, cooked and drained of grease
- 4 oz softened cream cheese
- 1 large egg
- 2 large cloves garlic, minced
- 1 tbsp chopped chives
- ½ tsp Italian seasoning
- ½ tsp salt

Instructions

1. Preheat oven to 350 degrees F.
2. In a medium bowl, whip the cream cheese with a hand mixer on low speed.
3. Mix the chives, garlic, salt, and Italian seasoning into the cream cheese and egg mixture.
4. Add the cheddar cheese, heavy cream, and water into the mixture. Mix with the hand mixer.
5. While using the hand mixer, slowly add almond flour into the mixture.
6. With a rubber spatula, fold the cooked sausage into the resulting dough mixture.

7. Drop the dough mixture into 8 wells of a muffin top pan, lightly greased, and forming a heaping mound in each.
8. Put in the oven and bake for 25 minutes.
9. Remove from the oven and let it cool before serving.

Breakfast Frittata with Fried Avocado and Black Olives

Cooking Time: 10 minutes
Calories: 599
Servings: 2

Ingredients
- 4 large eggs
- 1 avocado, peeled and sliced into thick slices
- 10 kalamata olives, pitted
- 2 oz full fat Brie cheese, thinly sliced
- 2 tbsp coconut or MCT oil
- 2 tbsp grass-fed butter
- 1 tsp Herbes de Provence
- ½ tsp salt

Instructions
1. In a large bowl, crack the eggs and whisk. Mix in the oils, Herbes de Provence, olives, and salt. Whisk until frothy.
2. Heat a large skillet to high. Melt the butter on it until it foams. Fry the avocado in the skillet until you get all sides slightly golden. Remove from the pan and set aside.
3. With the heat still on high, pour in the egg mixture into the skillet.
4. Place the brie cheese slices on the egg mixture
5. Cover the skillet and let it cook for around 3 minutes or when the bottom gets golden brown.
6. Flip the frittata with the help of lid or a plate and cook the other side for 2 minutes.
7. Serve on a large plate and top with the fried avocado.

Zucchini Breakfast Hash
Cooking Time: 15 minutes

Calories: 452
Servings: 1

Ingredients
- 2 slices of bacon, sliced
- 1 large egg
- 1 medium zucchini, diced into medium pieces
- ½ small white onion or a clove of garlic, peeled and finely chopped
- 1 tbsp coconut oil
- 1 tbsp freshly chopped chives or parsley
- ¼ tsp Himalayan pink salt

Instructions
1. Heat a frying pan on medium heat and grease with the coconut oil.
2. Sauté the onion on the pan. When it starts to sweat, add the bacon and continue sautéing until bacon is lightly browned.
3. Add the zucchini to the pan and briefly toss around the pan to soak in the juices. Cook for 10 to 15 minutes.
4. Remove from the heat and add the chopped chives or parsley.

5. Fry the egg with coconut oil and top it on dish to serve.

Fisherman's Eggs
Cooking Time: 10 minutes
Calories: 419
Servings: 1

Ingredients
- 2 large eggs
- 56 grams of sardines in olive oil
- ½ cup arugula
- 2.5 tbsp marinated artichoke hearts
- A pinch of salt
- Freshly ground black pepper to taste

Instructions
1. Preheat the oven to 375 degrees F.
2. Put the sardines on an oven-proof ceramic au gratin.
3. Break the eggs on top of the placed sardines.
4. Add arugula and artichokes on top.
5. Season with salt and pepper.
6. Put it in the oven for 10 minutes or until eggs reach your desired doneness.

7. Serve immediately.

Roasted Tomato Shakshuka

Cooking Time: 40 minutes
Calories: 612
Servings: 2

Ingredients
- 4 large eggs
- 1 large yellow onion, chopped
- 1 red bell pepper, sliced into strips
- 1.5 lb cherry tomatoes or small heirloom tomatoes, cut in half
- 2 fresh thyme sprigs, without leaves and finely chopped
- ¼ cup extra virgin olive oil
- 1 tbsp parsley, finely chopped
- ½ tbsp. cumin seeds
- 1 pinch cayenne
- Salt to taste

Instructions
1. Preheat oven to 350 degrees F.
2. Lightly oil a baking sheet and lay the tomatoes on it.
3. Sprinkle with salt.

4. Put it in the oven for 30 minutes or until tomatoes become soft and caramelized.
5. Heat a large deep pan and heat the cumin seeds on it. This would take at least a minute.
6. Add the olive oil into the pan and let it heat up before turning down the heat to low. Then, add the chopped onions for sautéing.
7. Add the pepper, thyme, parsley, and tomatoes. Sprinkle with salt and cayenne pepper.
8. When the contents of the pan is bubbling, break the eggs while making sure that they spread evenly in it.
9. Adjust the flame to its lowest setting and let it cook for at least 10 minutes or until the egg is cooked sunny-side up (egg white is set but yolk is soft).
10. Serve on separate plate while hot.

Green Buttered Eggs
Cooking Time: 8 minutes
Calories: 360
Servings: 1

Ingredients

- 4 large eggs
- 2 cloves of garlic, peeled and finely chopped
- ½ cup fresh parsley, chopped
- ½ cup fresh cilantro, chopped
- 1 tbsp coconut oil
- 1 tsp fresh thyme leaves
- ½ tsp salt
- ¼ tsp ground cumin
- ¼ tsp ground cayenne

Instructions

1. Heat a skillet on medium heat and melt the butter and coconut oil. This would take about at least a minute.
2. Set the flame to low and sauté the garlic until it starts to brown
3. Add cilantro and parsley to the pan and increase heat to medium. Wait for the two ingredients to crisp before proceeding to the next step.
4. Crack the eggs and add them to the pan without breaking the yolk
5. Cover the pan with a lid and decrease heat to low. Let it cook for at least 3 minutes

and it's done depending on your desired doneness for eggs.
6. Serve while hot. This is a good dish to serve with breakfast sausages.

Breakfast Sausage

Cooking Time: 15 minutes
Calories: 712
Servings: 2

Ingredients
- 1 lb ground pork
- 1 tbsp parmesan cheese
- 2 tsp cayenne pepper
- 1 ½ tsp salt
- 1 ½ tsp garlic powder
- 1 ½ tsp onion powder
- 1 tsp sage
- 1 tsp paprika
- ½ tsp nutmeg
- ½ tsp ground ginger

Instructions
1. Break the ground pork into a bowl and mix it well with all the other ingredients.

2. Form the mixture into patties of your desired size.
3. Heat a skillet on medium-high heat and grease with a bit of olive oil (just enough to coat the cooking surface).
4. Cook on both sides until there's no pinkish hue visible.
5. For thicker patties, finish it off in the oven at 300 degrees F for around 8 minutes. Avoid drying the patties out.

Chapter 5
Whole Food Lunch Ketogenic Recipes

Simple Olive Oil Dressing
Prep Time: 3 minutes
Calories: 42
Servings: 4

Ingredients
- 3 tbsp. extra virgin olive oil
- 1 tbsp. apple cider vinegar
- Pinch of Himalayan salt
- Dash of freshly ground black pepper

Instructions
1. Combine all the ingredients in a mixing bowl.
2. Whisk until ingredients are mixed.

3. Store in a container or toss it in a salad for four.

Keto Ranch Dressing

Prep Time: 3 minutes
Calories: 175
Servings: 4

Ingredients
- 1 cup almond milk
- ¼ cup unsalted sunflower seeds
- ¼ cup freshly squeezed lemon juice
- 1 clove of garlic
- 1 tbsp. minced fresh parsley
- 1 tbsp. dried chives
- 1 tbsp. chia seeds
- 2 tsp minced red onion
- 1 tsp aminos, coconut or Braggs
- 1 tsp mustard
- ¼ tsp celery seed

Instructions
1. Blend all the ingredients, except the parsley and chives, in a blender for 2 minutes until you get a smooth consistency.

2. Mix in the parsley and chives.
3. Store in a resealable container and refrigerate. Best served after overnight refrigeration.

Keto Caesar Dressing

Prep Time: 3 minutes
Calories: 288
Servings: 4

Ingredients

- 8 anchovy fillets, approx. 50g
- 2 cloves of garlic
- ¼ cup extra-virgin coconut oil
- ¼ cup extra-virgin olive oil
- 2 tbsp. mayonnaise
- 2 tbsp. freshly squeezed lemon juice
- 1 tbsp. apple cider vinegar
- 1 tbsp. mustard
- A pinch of Himalayan salt
- Freshly ground black pepper to taste

Instructions

1. Put all the ingredients in a blender and blend it on high for about a minute or until a smooth consistency is achieved.

2. Store in an airtight container. Dressing would last for a maximum of 5 days.

Tzatziki Sauce

Prep Time: 5 minutes
Calories: 270
Servings: 1

Ingredients
- 170g English cucumber, grated
- 8 oz. full-fat Greek yogurt
- 2 cloves of garlic, peeled and crushed
- 2 tsp extra-virgin olive oil
- 1 tsp. Himalayan salt

Instructions
1. In a strainer, mix together the cucumber and salt. Leave in the refrigerator overnight for the water to strain.
2. The next day, press any leftover water from the grated cucumber.
3. In a medium bowl, mix together the ingredients.
4. Store in an airtight container and refrigerate overnight for the flavors to

incorporate together. Serve with your salad or grilled fish or meat.

Basil Salad Dressing
Prep Time: 3 minutes
Calories: 289
Servings: 5

Ingredients
- 2 oz fresh basil
- ¾ cup extra-virgin olive oil
- 1 tsp freshly squeezed lemon juice
- ½ tsp sea salt
- ½ tsp freshly ground black pepper

Instructions
1. Blend all the ingredients in a blender until smooth.
2. Store in an airtight container and refrigerate to preserve. Serve with salad or your choice of keto noodles or pasta.

Cilantro Lime Dressing
Prep Time: 3 minutes
Calories: 327
Servings: 2

Ingredients
- Juice from 1 lime
- ½ of jalapeno pepper
- 1/3 cup of hemp oil
- ½ cup of fresh cilantro
- 1 clove of garlic
- A pinch of salt

Instructions
1. Blend all the ingredients until smooth.
2. Store in an airtight container and refrigerate to preserve. Serve with your favorite salad greens.

Green Keto Dressing

Prep Time: 3 minutes
Calories: 275
Servings: 3

Ingredients
- 1 cup fresh basil
- ¼ cup water
- ¼ cup extra-virgin olive oil
- 1 medium-sized avocado
- 1 clove of garlic
- 1 piece of capers

- 2 tbsp. hemp hearts
- 2 tbsp. red wine vinegar
- 2 tbsp. fresh chives
- 1 tbsp. white wine vinegar
- A pinch of sea salt
- A pinch of freshly ground black pepper

Instructions
1. Blend all the ingredients in a blender until smooth. Add more water by ¼ cup increments to make a thinner consistency, if desired.
2. Store in an airtight container and refrigerate to preserve. Serve with your favorite salad greens or simply as a deep for vegetables.

Bacon Mustard Dressing
Prep Time: 5 minutes
Calories: 360
Servings: 1

Ingredients
- 3 tbsp. of bacon grease
- 1 tbsp. red wine vinegar

- 1 tbsp. Dijon mustard
- 1 tsp chopped shallots
- ¼ tsp Stevia
- Salt and freshly ground black pepper to taste

Instructions
1. Whisk together the mustard and the vinegar.
2. While whisking add the other ingredients.
3. Top it on your favorite salad greens.

Chicken, Bacon, Avocado Caesar Salad
Prep Time: 5 minutes
Calories: 341
Servings: 4

Ingredients
- 1 ripe avocado, 1 inch slices
- 1 cup bacon, crumpled
- 1 chicken breast, grilled and sliced
- 3 tbsp. Ketogenic Caesar Dressing
- Lettuce, depending on amount preferred

Instructions

1. In a bowl or two, combine the avocado, chicken breast, and crumpled bacon.
2. Top with Caesar dressing and toss lightly
3. Toss with preferred amount of lettuce for a bigger meal

Cheese Pizza Rolls

Cooking Time: 30 minutes
Calories: 474
Servings: 1

Ingredients

- 2 cups mozzarella cheese
- ½ cup crumbled sausage, cooked
- ¼ cup chopped green and red peppers
- ¼ cup pizza sauce, sugar-free and carb-free
- 1 small tomato, sliced
- 1 tbsp. chopped white onions
- 1 tsp pizza seasoning

Instructions

1. Preheat oven to 400 degrees F.

2. Line a baking sheet with parchment paper and lightly grease it with olive oil.
3. Sprinkle a single-layer of cheese on the parchment paper-lined baking sheet. There should be no holes in the layer of cheese.
4. Sprinkle the pizza seasoning over the cheese.
5. Put it in the oven and let it bake for 20 minutes or until browned.
6. Remove from oven and test the cheese for doneness by gently sliding a silicone spatula at the edges and at the middle. If you're able to do so, proceed to the next step. If not, put it back in the oven until you're able to do so.
7. Add sausage, onions, peppers, and tomato on the cheese. Drizzle the tomato sauce on top of the toppings and cheese.
8. Put it back in the oven and let it cook for 10 minutes.
9. With the silicone spatula, check again that there parchment paper is not sticking to the cheese.
10. Slice the pizza vertically. This would usually give you 6 strips.

11. Let it cool then roll from top to bottom. Serve.

Broccoli Alfredo Fried Pizza
Cooking Time: 20 minutes
Calories: 435
Servings: 2

Ingredients
- 1 cup shredded mozzarella and cheddar cheese blend, equal parts
- 1 cup shredded mozzarella cheese
- 1/3 cup steamed and chopped broccoli heads
- ¼ cup mascarpone cheese
- 2 tbsp ghee
- 1 tbsp. heavy cream
- 1 tsp minced garlic
- 1/8 tsp lemon pepper seasoning
- 2 pinches salt
- Shaved asiago cheese to taste

Instructions
For the crust:

1. Heat a medium frying pan to medium heat. Add olive oil.

2. Once the oil is hot and shimmering, add the mozzarella and cheddar cheese blend by forming a circle in the pan.
3. Add the mozzarella cheese on top of the circle of cheese from the previous step.
4. Let it cook for around 5 minutes or until the cheese gets crispy and a spatula can easily slide under the edges. Carefully remove it from the pan with the help of the spatula. Let it cool on a plate.

For the toppings:

1. On the hot pan, add garlic, mascarpone cheese, ghee, heavy cream, lemon pepper, and salt.
2. Once it is melted and begins to bubble, immediately remove from the heat.
3. Drizzle half of the mixture over the crust.
4. Add the broccoli to the other half and cook for around a minute. Once the mixture is hot and bubbling, it's done.
5. Add the mixture to the pizza.
6. Sprinkle shaved asiago cheese. Optional, sprinkle extra lemon pepper seasoning. Serve.

Mushroom and Walnut Cauliflower Grits

Cooking Time: 25 minutes
Calories: 532
Servings: 3

Ingredients

- 6 oz. baby Portobello mushrooms, sliced
- 1 cup half and half
- 1 cup shredded sharp cheddar
- ½ cup water
- ½ cup chopped walnuts
- 3 cloves of garlic, minced
- 1 medium cauliflower
- 2 tbsp. butter
- 2 tbsp. olive oil
- 1 tbsp. smoked paprika
- 1 tbsp. rosemary
- Salt to taste

Instructions

1. Preheat oven to 400 degrees F. Line a baking sheet with foil.
2. In a bowl, combine the mushrooms, garlic, walnuts, rosemary, and smoked

paprika. Drizzle with olive oil and toss to coat everything with the oil.
3. Spread the combined ingredients on the foil-lined baking sheet. Season with salt and roast in the oven for 15 minutes.
4. Finely process one head of cauliflower florets in the food processor.
5. Transfer the processed cauliflower to a medium pot. Cover it with half a cup of water, heat it to medium heat, and let it steam for 5 minutes or until the cauliflower becomes slightly tender.
6. Reduce the heat to low then stir in the cheese and butter until the mixture is well combined and creamy. Season with salt to taste. For runny grits, add ¼ cup of water.
7. Once the mushrooms are soft and its edges are deep brown, remove the baking sheet and its contents from the oven.
8. Transfer the cauliflower grits to a bowl and top with the mushroom mixture. You can add extra butter if you want. Serve while hot.

Cauliflower Crust Pizza

Cooking Time: 30 minutes
Calories: 396
Servings: 2

Ingredients:
- 2 cups riced cauliflower
- 1 cup shredded parmesan cheese
- 1 cup shredded mozzarella cheese
- 1 egg, beaten
- 2 tsp Italian seasoning
- 1 tsp garlic powder
- ½ tsp garlic salt

Instructions:

To make riced cauliflower:
1. Cut off everything but the stem of the cauliflower.
2. Process it in a food processor or blender for a few seconds.
3. Microwave for 10 minutes.
4. Spread out the processed cauliflower on paper towels to drain it out of moisture. Pat it with paper towels to drain it even

further. Otherwise, you'll end up with a soggy crust.
5. You should have 2 cups worth of riced cauliflower.
6. Put it in a bowl and into the refrigerator to cool it down.

For the Pizza:

1. Preheat the oven to 450 degrees F
2. Mix together the cooled-down riced cauliflower, beaten egg, and half of the shredded parmesan in a bowl.
3. Add Italian seasoning, garlic salt, and garlic powder and mix.
4. Pour the mixture onto a baking sheet. You can either form a single crust or several smaller pizza crusts.
5. Put it in the oven for 15 to 20 minutes. It would take lesser time for smaller crusts. Take it out of the oven when the crust starts to get a golden brown color.
6. Top it off with the rest of the mozzarella cheese and your preferred sauce with toppings.

7. Put it back in the oven with the broil setting turned on. This would take at least 3 minutes depending on the sauce and toppings you put.
8. Let it cool for a bit then serve.

Oven Roasted Caprese Salad

Cooking Time: 30 minutes
Calories: 513
Servings: 3

Ingredients

- 4 cups baby spinach leaves
- 3 cups grape tomatoes
- ¼ cup fresh basil leaves
- 4 cloves of garlic, peeled
- 10 pieces of pearl sized mozzarella balls
- 2 tbsp avocado oil
- 1 tbsp pesto
- 1 tbsp brine reserved from the mozzarella cheese

Instructions

1. Preheat oven to 400 degrees F.

2. Line a baking sheet with foil and evenly spread out the garlic cloves and grape tomatoes on it.
3. Drizzle the garlic cloves and grape tomatoes with avocado oil. Toss it around to coat evenly. Put it in the oven for 20 to 30 minutes or until the ingredients release their juices and gain a slightly browned top.
4. Mix the brine with the pesto.
5. Put the spinach into a large serving bowl and top it with the tomatoes and garlic. Drizzle it with the brine and pesto sauce.
6. Add mozzarella balls and torn basil leaves. Serve.

Italian Cheesy Bread

Cooking Time: 20 minutes
Calories: 451
Servings: 4

Ingredients
- 1 ¼ cup shredded Monterey Jack
- 4 small slices Italian dry salami
- ¼ cup mild pepper rings

- 1 large egg
- 1 large egg yolk
- 4 tbsp. coconut flour
- 3 tbsp. flax seed meal
- 4 small slices provolone cheese
- 1 oz spinach leaves
- 1 tsp olive oil
- 1 tsp. Italian seasoning

Instructions

1. Preheat oven to 400 degrees F.
2. In a small bowl, combine flax seed meal, coconut flour, and seasoning together.
3. In a larger bowl, put the Monterey jack cheese and put it in the microwave for around a minute. You would want the shreds fully melted together.
4. Let the cheese rest at room temperature for about a minute then add the egg. Combine together.
5. Add the contents of the smaller bowl to the egg and cheese mix together. Keep mixing until the cheese fully incorporates the flour into the mixture forming a dough.

6. Lay out a piece of parchment paper then place the cheese dough on it. Place another sheet of parchment paper on top of it then, with a rolling pin, spread it out to a long shape with a width enough for the fillings in the middle and the braids surrounding the fillings.
7. Lay out the cheese and salami on the middle of the spread out dough.
8. Tear the spinach leaves then set those on the cheese and salami. Lay on the mild pepper rings on top then drizzle the fillings with the olive oil.
9. With a knife, cut diagonal strips on the sides of the dough. Fold up the ends of the dough while forming braids on top of the fillings.
10. Whisk the egg yolk. Brush on the dough.
11. Put it into the preheated oven then bake for 15 to 20 minutes. Once the braid gets a golden brown color, it is done.
12. Slice into four pieces. Serve.

Salmon Patties with Fresh Herbs

Cooking Time: 8 minutes
Calories: 487
Servings: 5

Ingredients

- 2 15 oz canned pink salmon flakes
- 4 oz pork rinds, crushed
- 2 large eggs
- ½ cup almond flour
- ¼ cup chopped fresh dill
- ¼ cup grated Parmesan
- 2 tbsp. chopped fresh chives
- 2 tbsp. olive oil
- 1 tsp. lemon zest
- Salt and pepper to taste

Keto Tartar Sauce:

- ½ cup mayonnaise
- 1 tbsp. diced dill pickle
- 1 tsp lemon juice
- 1 tsp finely diced green onion
- ½ tsp dill weed

Instructions

1. Open the cans of pink salmon and drain it of its liquid. Put it in a large mixing bowl.
2. Add the chives, parmesan cheese, dill, pork rinds, large eggs, lemon zest, and salt into the bowl with the salmon. Mix together thoroughly.
3. Form the mixture into 3 oz balls then flatten each into a patty with your palm. The mixture would give you around a total of 10 patties.
4. Put almond flour on a plate and dip both sides of each patty into it. Be careful of the patties as they are quite fragile and could break up easily.
5. Preheat a skillet to medium-high heat then grease it with the olive oil. Once the oil shimmers, fry the patties for a few minutes on each side. Once each side gets browned, it is fully cooked.
6. Mix together the ingredients of the tartar sauce.
7. Serve two patties for each serving with the tartar sauce and pair it with

vegetables; blanched broccoli and/or asparagus is recommended.

Sesame Tofu and Eggplant "Noodles"
Cooking Time: 15 minutes
Calories: 492
Servings: 3

Ingredients
- 1 lb block firm tofu
- 1 cup chopped cilantro
- ¼ cup sesame seeds
- ¼ cup soy sauce
- 1 whole eggplant (450 to 500 grams), peeled and julienned
- 3 tbsp rice vinegar
- 4 tbsp toasted sesame oil
- 2 cloves of garlic, finely minced
- 1 tsp crushed red pepper flakes
- 2 tsp Swerve
- 1 tbsp olive oil
- Salt and pepper to taste

Instructions
1. Preheat oven to 200 degrees F.

2. Wrap the tofu with paper towels and place it on a plate and place another plate on top of it. Weigh the top of it with about a pound to press the water out of it.
3. In a large mixing bowl, combine ¼ cup of the cilantro, rice vinegar, sesame oil, garlic, red pepper flakes, Swerve. Whisk together. Mix the eggplant with the marinade.
4. Heat a skillet on medium-low heat. Add the olive oil and cook the eggplant in its marinade until it gets soft. If the eggplant sticks, add sesame oil or olive oil.
5. Put the eggplant noodles into an oven safe dish. Cover it with foil. Turn off oven and put in the dish with the eggplant noodles.
6. Wipe the skillet of any leftover liquids and heat it back up over medium-low heat.
7. Unwrap the tofu and slice it into eight portions. Spread sesame seeds on a

plate and press the top and bottom sides of the tofu slice into the seeds.
8. Drop 2 tbsp of sesame oil on the skillet and fry the sesame-pressed sides of the tofu for 5 minutes on each side or until it begins to crisp up.
9. Pour the soy sauce into the skillet and have it coat the pieces of tofu. Cook until the soy sauce caramelizes the tofu.
10. Remove the dish of eggplant "noodles" from the oven and plate the tofu on top. Serve.

Keto Okonomiyaki
Cooking Time: 15 minutes
Calories: 692
Servings: 1

Ingredients
For the batter:

- 1 large egg
- 1 tbsp. softened butter
- 1 tbsp softened cream cheese
- 2 tbsp almond flour
- 1 tbsp flax meal

- ½ tsp baking powder
- ¼ tsp salt

For the filling:

- 3 oz shredded green cabbage
- 2 slices bacon, thickly sliced

For the toppings:

- ¼ cup mayonnaise
- 1 ½ tbsp. sugar-free barbeque sauce
- 1 tbsp bonito flakes
- ½ tbsp. seaweed flakes
- 1 tsp unseasoned rice vinegar

Instructions

1. In a small bowl, mix the mayonnaise and rice vinegar together.
2. In another bowl, mix the butter, cream cheese, almond flour, flax meal, baking powder, and salt until a smooth batter is formed.
3. Crack the egg and add it to the batter then stir until it is fully incorporated into the batter.
4. Mix and thoroughly coat the cabbage into the batter.

5. Preheat the skillet over medium heat and fry the bacon slices.
6. Flip the bacon after it crisps up. Arrange the bacon pieces on a tight circle in the center. Add a little olive oil if you're using a skillet that's is not non-stick.
7. Spread the batter over the bacon and use a silicone spatula to form a pancake. Cover with a lid and let it cook for around 5 to 7 minutes.
8. Once the bottom is browned, loosed up the edges with a spatula and flip over to its other side. Add more oil, if needed. Cover again with a lid and let it cook for 5 to 7 minutes.
9. Once done, transfer to a plate and spread the BBQ sauce on top of it. Drizzle the mayonnaise and rice vinegar on top and sprinkle the top with seaweed and bonito flakes.
10. Cut the pancake into quarters. Serve.

Quick Keto Egg Drop Soup
Cooking Time: 15 minutes

Calories: 243
Servings: 1

Ingredients
- 1 ½ cup chicken broth
- ½ cube chicken bouillon
- 2 large eggs
- 1 tbsp. butter
- 1 tsp chili garlic paste

Instructions
1. Get a pan and put it over the stove on medium-high heat.
2. Add the chicken broth, chicken bouillon, and butter into the pan. Bring it to a boil while stirring the contents together.
3. Add chili garlic paste then stir. Once the mixture starts to boil, turn off the stove.
4. Beat the eggs in a bowl and pour into the hot broth while stirring.
5. Let it sit for a few seconds to cook. Serve.

Crispy Tofu and Bok-Choy Salad
Cooking Time: 30 minutes
Calories: 549

Servings: 2

Ingredients

For the Oven-Baked Tofu:

- 15 oz. Extra firm Tofu
- 1 tbsp Soy Sauce
- 1 tbsp Sesame Oil
- 1 tbsp Water
- 1 tsp Minced Garlic
- 1 tbsp Rice Wine Vinegar
- Juice from ½ a lemon

Bok-Choy Salad:

- 9 oz Bok-Choy, chopped into small slices
- 1 stalk Green Onion
- 3 tbsp coconut oil
- 1 tbsp. cilantro, chopped
- 1 tbsp. sambal olek
- 1 tbsp. peanut butter
- Juice from ½ a lemon
- 7 drops Stevia

Instructions

1. Place the tofu on a plate and place another plate on top of it. Put a weight

of about a pound to press it dry. This would take around 5 to 6 hours.
2. Combine soy sauce, sesame oil, garlic, vinegar, water, and lemon juice to make the marinade.
3. Chop the dried out tofu into squares and place in a bag with the marinade. Let it marinade for at least 30 minutes to overnight.
4. Preheat oven to 350 degrees F. Line a baking sheet with parchment paper and place tofu on it. Bake for 30 minutes.
5. Mix all the salad ingredients aside from bok-choy to make the dressing.
6. Remove tofu from oven and assemble it with the bok-choy and sauce. Serve.

Brie and Apple Crepes
Cooking Time: 10 minutes
Calories: 495
Servings: 3

Ingredients
For the Crepe Batter:

- 4 large eggs

- 4 oz cream cheese
- ½ tsp baking soda
- ¼ tsp sea salt

For the Toppings:

- 4 oz brie cheese, room temperature and thinly sliced
- 2 oz chopped pecans
- 1 small gala apple, thinly sliced.
- 1 tbsp. unsalted butter
- ¼ tsp ground cinnamon
- Fresh mint leaves, for garnish

Instructions
1. Blend all the crepe batter ingredients in a blender until smooth.
2. Heat a bit of butter on a pan over medium heat.
3. Ladle enough of the batter on the pan to create a thin and evenly spread out crepe. Cook for about 2 to 3 minutes or until the top looks dry. Gently flip it to the other side with a large spatula and let it cook for a few seconds.
4. Repeat the steps until you run out of batter or until you get 12 crepes. Layer

the crepes on top of each other on a plate.
5. In a small pan, melt a tablespoon of butter and toast the pecans until it becomes fragrant. Avoid browning the pecans too much. Sprinkle with cinnamon then mix. Transfer to a plate and let it cool.
6. Arrange the brie and apple slices on a crepe and top it with some pecans. Repeat on the other crepes you made until all toppings have been used.
7. Garnish with mint. Serve it flat or rolled on plate.

Low-Carb Guacamole

Prep Time: 15 minutes
Calories: 589
Servings: 2

Ingredients
- 3 avocadoes, mashed
- 6 grape tomatoes, diced
- 1 lime
- 1 clove of garlic
- ¼ cup diced red onion

- 1 tbsp. olive oil
- ¼ tsp salt
- 1/8 tsp freshly ground black pepper
- 1/8 tsp crushed red pepper
- Fresh cilantro, amount varies on preference

Instructions
1. Combine and mix the mashed avocadoes, diced tomatoes, and diced red onions.
2. Crush the garlic clove into the mix.
3. Add olive oil and mix.
4. Add cilantro and squeeze out the juice of the lime into the mix.
5. Season with salt, pepper, and red pepper. You can skip the red pepper if you prefer.
6. Mix well and serve. Can be paired with another dish or served solo.

Chipotle Steak Bowl
Cooking Time: 8 minutes
Calories: 585
Servings: 4

Ingredients
- 1 serving Low Carb Guacamole (see previous recipe)
- 16 oz skirt steak
- 4 oz pepper jack cheese, shredded
- 1 cup sour cream
- 1 handful of fresh cilantro
- 1 splash Chipotle Tabasco Sauce (optional)
- Salt and Pepper to taste

Instructions
1. Preheat a skillet, preferably cast iron, to high heat.
2. Rub the skirt steak with salt and pepper. Once the skillet is very hot, cook it for 3 to 4 minutes on each side. Let the skirt steak rest on a plate.
3. Make the low-carb guacamole according to instructions.
4. Once the steak has been rested for at least ten minutes, slice it against the grain into thin strips. You would get 4 portions out of a 16 oz steak.
5. Top the skirt steak slices with shredded pepper jack cheese.

6. Top each portion of the steak with a quarter of the guacamole and followed by a quarter of the sour cream.
7. Splash with Chipotle Tabasco Sauce and garnish with fresh cilantro. Serve.

Chicken Salad Stuffed Avocado

Cooking Time: 40 minutes
Calories: 578
Servings: 1

Ingredients

- 1 medium avocado, pitted
- 3 oz chicken breast
- 1/3 cup sour cream
- 1 stalk celery, chopped
- 1 tbsp. red onion, diced

Instructions

1. Cook chicken breast on low heat. Shred the meat by using two forks.
2. Combine the chicken, red onion, and celery in a bowl.
3. Scoop half of the pitted avocado and add it to the bowl of chicken mixture.
4. Add sour cream and season it with salt and pepper to taste.

5. Toss the chicken salad and scoop it on top of the other half of the avocado. Serve.

Quick Keto Smoothie Bowl
Prep Time: 5 minutes
Calories: 706
Servings: 1

Ingredients
- 1 cup spinach
- ½ cup almond milk
- 4 raspberries
- 4 walnuts
- 1 scoop low-carb protein powder
- 2 tbsp. heavy cream
- 1 tbsp. coconut oil
- 1 tbsp. unsweetened shredded coconut
- 1 tsp chia seeds
- 2 ice cubes

Instructions
1. Blend the spinach, almond milk, heavy cream, coconut oil, and ice in a blender. The mixture should be thoroughly

combined and have an even consistency.
2. Pour the smoothie in a bowl.
3. Top it with the remaining ingredients and mix. Serve.

Feta and Pesto Omelette
Cooking Time: 10 minutes
Calories: 514
Servings: 1

Ingredients
- 1 oz feta cheese
- 3 large eggs
- 2 fresh tomatoes of your choice, sliced
- 1 tbsp. grass-fed butter
- 1 tbsp. heavy cream
- 1 tbsp. pesto
- Salt and pepper to taste

Instructions
1. Beat the eggs in a bowl with the heavy cream.
2. On a frying pan, heat the butter over medium heat. Pour in the eggs.

3. When the eggs are almost done, sprinkle ¾ of the feta cheese onto half of the omelette. Spread the pesto on top of the feta cheese.
4. Fold the bare half of the omelette over the half with the pesto and feta cheese. Let it cook for 4 to 5 minutes to melt the cheese.
5. Take it off the pan and transfer on a plate. Garnish with the remaining feta cheese and more basil if you want. Serve with the sliced fresh tomatoes on the side.

Spiced Pumpkin Soup

Cooking Time: 25 minutes
Calories: 588
Servings: 4

Ingredients

- 1 ½ cup chicken broth
- 1 cup pumpkin puree
- ½ cup heavy cream
- 4 slices of bacon
- 2 cloves of roasted garlic, minced

- 1 bay leaf
- ¼ medium onion, chopped
- 4 tbsp. butter
- 2 tbsp. chopped fresh parsley
- 2 tbsp. sour cream
- ½ tsp salt
- ½ tsp pepper
- ½ tsp ginger, freshly minced
- ¼ tsp coriander
- ¼ tsp cinnamon
- 1/8 tsp nutmeg

Instructions
1. In a saucepan, melt the butter over medium-low heat.
2. Once the butter turns a dark golden brown color, add the onions, garlic, and ginger. Cook for 2 to 3 minutes
3. Once the onions become translucent, add the spices and stir well. After a minute or two, add the pumpkin puree and chicken broth while stirring.
4. Bring the contents of the saucepan to a boil then turn the heat to low. Simmer the contents for 20 minutes. When the

20 minutes are up, blend the contents with an immersion blender until smooth.
5. Simmer for another 20 minutes.
6. In a frying pan, cook the slices of bacon and save 3 tbsp. of its grease.
7. After simmering the soup for 20 minutes, mix in the heavy cream and bacon grease.
8. Transfer to a bowl. Crumble the bacon on top of the soup, sprinkle the chopped parsley, and drizzle the sour cream. Serve.

Buffalo Chicken Soup
Cooking Time: 60 minutes
Calories: 758
Servings: 6

Ingredients
- 4 chicken breasts
- 2 carrots, small diced
- 4 stalks of celery, chopped
- 4 cups chicken broth
- 2 oz cream cheese

- ½ cup heavy cream
- 6 tbsp. grass-fed butter
- 1 tsp salt
- ½ tsp thyme
- ½ tsp cayenne
- Red hot sauce to taste

For garnish:
- Cold sour cream
- Bleu cheese
- Chopped green onion

Instructions

1. In an oiled pot over medium heat, cook the carrots and chopped celery stalks.
2. When the carrots and celery have broken down, place the chicken breasts to cook alongside the vegetables. Cover the pot.
3. Once the chicken breasts are cooked, take it out of the pot and shred it by using two forks. You can put it back in after shredding.
4. Pour the chicken broth into the pot and add the butter, cream cheese, and heavy cream into it.

5. When the contents of the pot come into a boil, put the shredded chicken breasts back in if you haven't done so.
6. Add the hot sauce, herbs, and cayenne. Simmer for 20 minutes.
7. Take it out of the heat and transfer to a bowl. Garnish the soup with the bleu cheese, cold sour cream, and green onion on top. Serve.

Split Pea and Ham Soup
Cooking Time: 60 minutes
Calories: 697
Servings: 6

Ingredients
- 8 cups chicken broth
- 4 cups split peas, rinsed
- 2 lbs. of ham, cubed into ½ inch pieces
- 4 carrots, chopped
- 2 white onions, chopped
- 8 cloves of garlic, finely chopped
- 4 tbsp. grass-fed butter
- 1 tbsp. salt
- 1 tbsp. thyme
- ½ parsley

- 1 tsp pepper
- ½ tsp cayenne

Instructions

1. Heat a frying pan over medium-high heat. Put some oil on it and brown the cubes of ham.
2. In a large oiled soup pot, cook the onions, carrots, and garlic.
3. When the onions become translucent, add the browned ham and pour the chicken broth over the ingredients. Bring to a boil.
4. Once the contents of the pot come to a boil, add in the split peas and stir. Let it come to a boil again then lower the heat to simmer.
5. Add in the herbs and spices and simmer the contents of the pot for an hour and a half.
6. Once the simmer is done, break down any peas that are still whole to make the soup thick.
7. Serve.

Keto Grilled Cheese Sandwich

Cooking Time: 10 minutes
Calories: 543
Servings: 1

Ingredients
- 2 large eggs
- 2 tbsp almond flour
- 2 tbsp soft butter
- 1 tbsp butter for frying
- 1 ½ tbsp. psyllium husk powder
- ½ tsp baking powder
- 2 oz cheddar cheese

Instructions
1. In a cup, mix together the soft butter, almond flour, husk powder, and baking powder until you form a thick dough.
2. Add the eggs and continue mixing until the dough thickens. This would take around a minute to achieve.
3. Pour the dough into a square bowl or container. Level the top and clean the sides.
4. Microwave for 90 to 100 seconds. Make sure it's done.

5. Flip the container on a plate and tap it on the bottom. This will remove the "bread" from the container. Cut the bread in half to make two equal slices.
6. Stick the cheddar cheese in between the two slices.
7. Heat a pan over medium heat and melt the butter on it. Add the sandwich to soak the butter into the "bread". Flip it to equally cook the butter in the other side of the sandwich. This would give the sandwich a crisp top and bottom.
8. Serve.

Chapter 6
Whole Food Dinner Ketogenic Recipes

Creamy Garlic Chicken

Cooking Time: 20 minutes
Calories: 445
Servings: 4

Ingredients
- 1 ½ lbs. boneless chicken breast, thinly sliced
- 1 cup heavy cream
- 1 cup chopped spinach
- ½ cup chicken broth
- ½ cup parmesan cheese
- ½ cup sun dried tomatoes
- 2 tbsp. olive oil

- 1 tsp garlic powder
- 1 tsp Italian seasoning

Instructions
1. In a large skillet, heat olive oil over medium-high heat. Cook the chicken breast for at least 3 minutes on each side. Remove chicken from skillet then set aside.
2. On the same skillet, add heavy cream, chicken broth, parmesan cheese, Italian seasoning and garlic powder. Whisk contents over the same level of heat in the previous step until it thickens.
3. Add spinach and sun dried tomatoes. Simmer until spinach wilts. Add chicken back into the skillet.
4. Serve.

Loaded Mashed "Potatoes"
Cooking Time: 8 minutes
Calories: 624
Servings: 2

Ingredients
- 1 lb cauliflower florets

- 1 cup grated cheddar cheese
- 4 oz sour cream
- 2 slices bacon, cooked and crumbled
- 3 tbsp butter
- 2 tbsp snipped chives
- ¼ tsp garlic powder
- Salt and pepper to taste

Instructions

1. Cut the cauliflower into florets then put in a microwave safe bowl and add tbsp of water. Cover with cling film
2. Microwave 5 to 8 minutes until cauliflower is tender. Take it out of the microwave, drain excess water, and let the contents sit uncovered for two minutes.
3. Process the cauliflower until fluffy. Add garlic powder, sour cream, and butter into the food processor. Process the contents until it has the consistency of mashed potatoes.
4. Transfer the contents to the bowl. Add most of the snipped chives. Season the contents.

5. Top the cauliflower with bacon and the remaining cheddar cheese and chives. Microwave or broil to melt the cheese. Serve.

Keto Salisbury Steak with Mushroom Gravy
Cooking Time: 30 minutes
Calories: 535
Servings: 6

Ingredients
For the Salisbury Steak:

- 2 lbs ground chuck (80/20 meat to fat ratio)
- ¾ cup almond flour
- ¼ cup beef broth
- 1 tbsp dried onion flakes
- 1 tbsp fresh parsley, chopped
- 1 tbsp Worcestershire sauce
- 1 ½ tsp salt
- ½ tsp garlic powder
- ½ freshly ground black pepper

For the Gravy:

- 2 cups sliced button mushrooms
- 1 cup sliced yellow onions
- ½ cup beef broth
- ¼ cup sour cream
- 4 tbsp butter
- ½ tbsp Worcestershire sauce
- Salt and pepper to taste

Instructions

For the Salisbury Steak:

1. Preheat oven to 375 degrees F.
2. In a medium sized bowl, combine all the steak ingredients and mix thoroughly.
3. Form ground chuck mixture into 1-inch thick oval patties. You would get around 6 of these patties.
4. Put the patties in a baking sheet and cook in the oven for 18 minutes.

For the gravy:

1. In a large skillet, melt half of the butter over medium heat.
2. Add mushrooms and cook it until it gets a golden brown color. Each side would take 2 minutes to cook.
3. Add onions. Cook for five minutes.

4. Add broth and Worcestershire sauce. Simmer for two minutes while stirring the contents and scraping of the glazed bit of the bottom of the skillet.
5. Add and stir into the mixture the sour cream. After stirring, transfer the gravy to a bowl. If you prefer thicker gravy, cook the mixture for a few more minutes.
6. Season it with salt and pepper.
7. Pour on top of the warm Salisbury Steaks. Serve.

Garlic Butter Brazilian Steak
Cooking Time: 15 minutes
Calories: 467
Servings: 4

Ingredients:
- 1 ½ lbs skirt steak, trimmed and cut into 4 slices
- 2 oz unsalted grass-fed butter
- 6 cloves of garlic, peeled
- 2 tbsp vegetable oil
- 1 tbsp chopped fresh flat-leaf parsley
- Salt and freshly ground pepper to taste

Instructions:
1. Smash the garlic cloves and light sprinkle it with salt. After doing so, mince the garlic cloves.
2. Pat the meat dry and generously season on both sides with salt and pepper.
3. In a 12-inch skillet, heat the oil on medium-high heat. Once the oil becomes shimmering hot, start browning the steak on both sides. This would take at least 2 minutes for each side to have the meat done medium rare.
4. Once done, transfer skirt steak to a plate and rest the meat.
5. In smaller skillet, melt the butter over low heat. Sauté the garlic until golden brown. Season lightly with salt.
6. Spoon the resulting garlic butter sauce over the steak and garnish it by sprinkling parsley on top. Serve.

Garlic Shrimp Noodles
Cooking Time: 5 minutes
Calories: 493

Servings: 1

Ingredients
- 2 medium-sized zucchini
- ¾ lb medium shrimp, peeled and deveined
- 4 cloves of garlic, minced
- 1 lemon, get juice and zest
- 1 tbsp olive oil
- Salt and pepper to taste
- Red pepper flakes to taste (optional)
- Chopped fresh parsley for garnish

Instructions
1. Spiralize zucchini and set aside.
2. On a skillet over medium heat, add olive oil and lemon juice and zest. Once it's warm enough, add the shrimp and cook for at least a minute on each side.
3. Add garlic and red pepper flakes. Cook and stir contents for another minute.
4. Add the spiralized zucchini and toss around the skillet for 2 to 3 minutes until slight cooked and softened.
5. Season with salt and pepper. Garnish with parsley. Serve while hot.

Blackened Salmon with Avocado Salsa

Cooking Time: 15 minutes
Calories: 519
Servings: 2

Ingredients

For the Blackened Salmon:

- 6 oz salmon, cut into 4 equal portions
- 1 tbsp olive oil
- 4 tsp Cajun seasoning

For the Avocado Salsa:

- 2 avocado, diced
- 1 jalapeno, finely diced
- ¼ cup red onion, diced
- 1 tbsp cilantro, chopped
- 1 tbsp lime juice
- Salt to taste

Instructions

1. Season and rub the salmon with Cajun seasoning
2. Over medium high-heat, heat oil in a skillet with a heavy bottom. Once hot, add seasoned salmon and cook until it

gets a color between deep golden brown and lightly charred on a few spots. Flip then repeat on the other side.
3. Mix all the ingredients for the avocado salsa.
4. Serve the salmon with the avocado salsa on the side.

Roasted Shrimp and Asparagus in Lemon, Butter, and Garlic

Cooking Time: 12 minutes
Calories: 578
Servings: 2

Ingredients

For the shrimp:

- 1 ½ lbs medium uncooked shrimp; peeled, deveined, and tails removed
- 3 garlic cloves, minced
- 3 tbsp chopped fresh parsley
- 3 tbsp grass-fed butter, cubed
- 1 ½ tbsp lemon juice
- 1 tbsp olive oil
- ½ tsp salt
- ¼ tbsp paprika

- 1/8 tsp pepper
- 1/8 tsp red pepper flakes

For the asparagus

- 1 lb thin asparagus, ends trimmed
- 1 garlic clove, minced
- 1 tbsp olive oil
- ¼ tsp salt
- 1/8 tsp pepper

Instructions

1. Preheat the oven to 400 degrees F.
2. Get a 10x15 inch Jelly Roll Pan and line it with foil. Lightly spray its surface with cooking spray.
3. Add the asparagus on foil-lined pan and drizzle with the tablespoon of olive oil. Add all the other ingredients for the asparagus and toss until asparagus gets an even coat. Put it in the oven and roast for 4 to 6 minutes.
4. Take out the pan from the oven and push all the asparagus to one side. Add shrimp on the vacant side and drizzle the ingredients (except the butter) for

the shrimp. Toss shrimp to get an even coating of ingredients on it.
5. Top the asparagus with a tablespoon of butter and the shrimp with 2 tablespoons of butter. Put the pan back in the oven and roast for 6 minutes or until shrimp gets an opaque appearance.
6. Remove the pan from the oven. Drizzle with lemon juice and season with additional salt and pepper to taste. Serve with cauliflower florets "rice".

Cashew Chicken

Cooking Time: 20 minutes
Calories: 552
Servings: 4

Ingredients

- 3 pieces skinless and boneless chicken thighs
- ¼ cup cashews
- ½ medium green bell pepper
- ¼ medium white onion
- 2 tbsp olive oil
- 1 ½ tbsp soy sauce

- 1 tbsp rice wine vinegar
- 1 tbsp minced garlic
- 1 tbsp sesame oil
- 1 tbsp sesame seeds
- 1 tbsp green onions
- ½ tbsp chili garlic sauce
- 1/2 tsp ground ginger
- Salt and pepper to taste

Instructions

1. Heat a frying pan on low heat. Once the pan is hot enough, toast the cashews for 8 minutes or until they develop a fragrant smell and a lightly brown color. Remove from the pan and set aside.
2. Dice the chicken. Slice the onion and pepper into equally-sized chunks.
3. Set the heat under the pan to high. Add olive oil
4. Once the oil is hot enough, add chicken thighs. Cooking time will be around 5 minutes.
5. Once chicken is cooked, add in onions, pepper, garlic, chili garlic sauce, ginger, salt, and pepper. Let the contents of the

pan cook for 2 to 3 minutes from the time the last ingredient was added.
6. Once the time is up, add the cashews, soy sauce, and rice wine vinegar. Cook on high to reduce the liquid to a sticky consistency.
7. Top with sesame seeds and drizzle with sesame oil. Serve.

Sausage Casserole
Cooking Time: 30 minutes
Calories: 474
Servings: 4

Ingredients
- 1 pound pork sausage
- 2 cups shredded green cabbage
- 2 cups diced zucchini
- 1 ½ cup shredded cheddar cheese
- ½ cup diced onion
- ½ cup mayonnaise
- 3 large eggs
- 2 tsp yellow mustard
- 1 tsp ground sage, preferably dried
- Cayenne pepper to taste

Instructions
1. Preheat the oven at 375 degrees F.
2. Brown sausage in skillet over medium heat and break the casing while moving it around the skillet. Continue browning until it is almost cooked
3. With the juices of the sausage, sauté zucchini and onion in the same skillet. Continue until vegetables become tender and sausage becomes thoroughly cooked
4. Remove from heat and put the mixture into a lightly greased casserole dish. Set aside.
5. Whisk eggs, mustard, mayonnaise, sage, and pepper. Keep whisking until you get a smooth mixture.
6. Mix a cup of the shredded cheese into the mixture.
7. Pour the mixture on top of the sausage and vegetables.
8. Top the casserole mixture with the leftover cheese.
9. Put the casserole in the oven and cook it for 30 minutes. The dish would be done

once the cheese is melted and lightly browned and there's bubbling on the edges of the dish.
10. Take it out of the oven and serve while hot. The whole dish gives you a total of 6 servings.

Ricotta Stuffed Salmon Rolls

Cooking Time: 25 minutes
Calories: 478
Servings: 2

Ingredients

- 4 pieces 5 oz salmon fillets with skin removed
- 1 oz ricotta
- ½ lb asparagus, trimmed
- ½ cup chicken broth
- ½ cup grated parmesan
- 2 tbsp chopped basil
- 2 tbsp lemon juice
- 1 tbsp butter
- 2 tsp lemon zest
- 2 tsp cornstarch
- Salt and pepper to taste

Instructions
1. Preheat the oven to 425 degrees F.
2. Season the salmon with salt and pepper. Lay skin side up on a baking sheet lined with parchment paper.
3. In a bowl, mix the ricotta, parmesan, basil, and lemon zest. Thoroughly mix the ingredients until the contents have an even consistency. Season with salt and pepper to taste then mix again thoroughly to combine well.
4. Divide the mixture into 5 portions and top each portion on top of the salmon fillets. Roll the fillets up.
5. Put the rolled up salmon fillets in the oven. Cooking will take around 15 to 20 minutes.
6. As the salmon fillets are cooking in the oven, dissolve the cornstarch in half of the chicken broth.
7. Heat a small saucepan over medium heat and melt the butter in it. Add in the rest of the chicken broth and the lemon juice. Stir well then add in the chicken broth and cornstarch mixture. Simmer

while stirring for 3 to 5 minutes or until you get a thickened sauce.
8. Once the salmons are cooked, take them out of the oven and put them in the plate. Top the fillets with the thickened sauce and garnish with lemon zest and parsley or basil (optional).

Keto Spaghetti ala Carbonara

Cooking Time: 10 minutes
Calories: 436
Servings: 4

Ingredients

- 680g Shiritaki noodles
- 5 oz thick-cut bacon, chopped
- 3 large eggs
- 2 large garlic cloves, minced
- 1 cup grated Parmesan
- 1 ½ tbsp butter
- Parsley, salt, and pepper to taste

Instructions

1. In a bowl, crack the eggs and beat it with ¾ of the grated parmesan.

2. Heat a deep pan over medium-high heat. Once it is hot enough, melt the butter on it.
3. Add the bacon and cook until crispy.
4. Add the minced garlic and lower the heat to medium-low.
5. Add the shirataki noodles into the pan.
6. Stir the noodles and coat it with the combined grease from the butter and the bacon.
7. Once the noodles become warm, take the pan off the heat and immediately add the egg and cheese mixture onto the noodles. Toss and mix the noodles to fully incorporate the egg and cheese mixture into it.
8. The eggs shouldn't scramble but become a thick sauce that coats the noodles.
9. Season with salt and pepper and toss the noodles some more.
10. Transfer to the plate and top with parsley and remaining parmesan cheese.

One Pot Shrimp Alfredo

Cooking Time: 15 minutes
Calories: 456
Servings: 3

Ingredients

- 1 lb raw shrimp; cleaned, deshelled, and deveined
- 4 oz cream cheese, cubed
- 5 whole sundried tomatoes, julienned
- ½ cup whole milk
- ½ cup shredded parmesan cheese
- ¼ cup baby kale
- 1 tbsp salted butter
- 1 tbsp garlic powder
- 1 tsp dried basil
- 1 tsp salt

Instructions

1. Melt the butter in a large skillet with the stovetop on medium heat.
2. Reduce the heat to medium low then add the shrimp to the skillet.
3. Sauté the shrimp for 3 minutes. Make sure to toss and turn around the shrimp in the skillet to prevent overcooking.

4. Once the shrimp gain a pinkish hue, add the cream cheese and milk into the skillet.
5. Increase the heat to medium while stirring until the cheese melts and there are no lumpy formations present.
6. Next, sprinkle the contents of the skillet with garlic, basil, and salt then stir it into the mixture very well.
7. Add the parmesan cheese and stir to combine. Simmer until the sauce thickens.
8. Fold in the sundried tomatoes and baby kale into the contents of the skillet.
9. Remove from heat and serve immediately while hot.

Eggplant Bacon Alfredo
Cooking Time: 30 minutes
Calories: 501
Servings: 5

Ingredients
- 1 ½ lbs eggplant, peeled and julienned
- 1 lb bacon, chopped
- 2 cloves of garlic

- 1 cup heavy cream
- 1 cup shredded parmesan
- 2 tbsp butter
- 1 tbsp lemon juice
- 1 tbsp white wine

Instructions

1. Fry the bacon in a large skillet over medium heat. Remove the bacon from the skillet once it renders and becomes crispy. Transfer bacon to a plate lined with paper towels.
2. Cook the julienned eggplant in bacon grease. It will soften and soak up the bacon grease on the skillet.
3. Create a well in the center of the pan and put in the butter. Stir the eggplant noodles to coat them with melted butter.
4. Add the grated garlic and mix it in the eggplant noodles.
5. Add the heavy cream, white wine, and lemon juice into the skillet then stir.
6. Add the parmesan cheese then mix.
7. Add half of the bacon into the contents of the skillet.

8. Transfer to a plate then top it with the remaining bacon. Garnish with fresh basil if desired. Serve.

Roasted Sea Bass with Herbed Cauliflower Salad

Cooking Time: 15 minutes
Calories: 689
Servings: 1

Ingredients
- 10 oz whole sea bass, scaled and cleaned
- 2 lemons
- 1 cup finely grated cauliflower
- 1/3 cup fresh flat leaf parsley
- 1/3 cup finely chopped fresh mint
- 1/3 cup green olives, finely chopped
- 3 tbsp extra virgin olive oil
- Salt and pepper to taste

Instructions
1. Preheat the oven to 400 degrees F.
2. Rub the sea bass with a tablespoon of extra virgin olive oil and place on a

baking sheet lined with parchment paper.
3. Thinly slice one lemon and stuff it with some of the herbs into the sea bass.
4. Cook the sea bass in the oven for around 15 minutes or until the thickest part of the fish looks cooked.
5. Zest and juice the remaining lemon.
6. Using a large bowl, mix together the olives, grated cauliflower, lemon zest, lemon juice, herbs, and the remaining extra virgin olive oil. Season the mixture with salt and pepper to taste.
7. Serve the sea bass along with the cauliflower salad.

Nacho Steak Skillet
Cooking Time: 40 minutes
Calories: 497
Servings: 4

Ingredients
- 8 oz beef round tip steak, sliced thinly
- 1 oz shredded cheddar cheese
- 1 oz shredded Monterey Jack cheese
- 140g avocado

- 30g canned jalapeno slices
- 1 lb cauliflower
- 1/3 cup coconut oil
- 1/3 cup sour cream
- 1 tbsp grass-fed butter
- 1 tsp chili powder
- ½ tsp turmeric

Instructions

1. Preheat the oven to 400 degrees F.
2. Discard the leaves and bottom stem of the cauliflower. Slice it across the head and break or chop it into chip-like shapes.
3. In a large mixing bowl, whisk together the refined coconut oil, turmeric, and chili powder. Then, add the cauliflower and toss to evenly coat the pieces.
4. On a baking sheet, spread thinly the cauliflower. Evenly season with salt and pepper. Cook it in the oven for at least 20 minutes.
5. While the cauliflower is roasting, preheat an oven-safe skillet (preferably cast iron) on medium-high heat.

6. Season both sides of the steak with salt and pepper.
7. Melt the butter on the skillet. Once the butter stops foaming, put in the steak. Just let it cook and avoid disturbing it. Then, flip the steak cook on the other side. Once done, remove from the pan and let it rest for at least 10 minutes.
8. After it's done, remove the cauliflower from the oven. Transfer it to the skillet you used for the stake and mix it around the skillet to soak up the leftover juices.
9. After resting it for 10 minutes, slice the steak into strips, preferably fork-sized.
10. Top the cauliflower on the skillet with the steak and, then, with the shredded cheddar and Monterey jack cheeses and the jalapenos.
11. Put the skillet in the oven and cook for 5 to 10 minutes or until the cheese melts.
12. Serve with guacamole, sour cream, and hot sauce on the side or mix it in.

Garnish with cilantro and green onion slices if desired.

Savory Italian Baked Egg

Cooking Time: 30 minutes
Calories: 529
Servings: 5

Ingredients
- 10 large eggs
- 12 oz broccoli florets
- 2 cups diced chicken breast, cooked
- 1 cup shredded extra sharp cheese
- ½ cup tomato sauce
- ½ cup heavy whipping cream
- ½ cup grated Parmesan
- 3 tbsp mustard
- 2 tsp garlic and herb seasoning
- 1 tsp parsley flakes

Instructions
1. Preheat oven to 350 degrees F.
2. In a large mixing bowl, crack the eggs and whisk.

3. Add the mustard, heavy whipping cream, and garlic and herb seasoning. Whisk very well.
4. Once mixed well, whisk into the mixture the tomato sauce until there are no lumps visible.
5. Add the chicken and broccoli then mix.
6. Grease a large baking pan or casserole dish and then pour in the mixture.
7. Sprinkle on top the parmesan cheese and, then, the parsley flakes.
8. Bake for 30 minutes or until the top forms a crust.
9. Once it's done, top the dish with the shredded sharp cheese. Serve.

Hasselback Marinara Chicken
Cooking Time: 35 minutes
Calories: 397
Servings: 6

Ingredients
- 3 whole chicken breasts
- 10 oz spinach
- 4 oz cream cheese
- 3 oz mozzarella slices

- 1/3 cup shredded mozzarella
- 1 tbsp olive oil
- Salt and pepper to taste
- Tomato sauce to taste

Instructions

1. Preheat the oven to 400 degrees F.
2. In a microwave safe bowl, place the spinach, cream cheese, and mozzarella. Microwave for 2 minutes or until the cheeses melt.
3. Mix the contents of the bowl then add salt and pepper to taste. This would be the chicken's cheese filling.
4. Place horizontal cuts across each chicken breast without slicing all the way through the meat. This would be where you would be stuffing the chicken with the filling.
5. Stuff the chicken in the cuts you made with the cheese filling.
6. Brush the bare surfaces of the chicken breasts with olive oil. Cook in the oven for 25 minutes or until the chicken reaches an internal temperature of 125 degrees F.

7. Take the chicken out and top with tomato sauce and the mozzarella slices.
8. Broil in the oven for 5 minutes or until the cheese melts and gets a hint of browning.
9. Serve.

Roasted Herbed Chicken with Brussels Sprouts Side

Cooking Time: 1 hour 20 minutes
Calories: 477
Servings: 8

Ingredients

- 5 lbs whole chicken for roasting, giblets removed
- 2 lbs Brussels Sprouts
- 1 whole lemon, pierced several times
- 1 small bunch fresh thyme
- 1 small bunch fresh oregano
- 4 tbsp softened butter
- 1 tbsp olive oil
- 1 tbsp dried parsley
- 1 tbsp dried marjoram
- Salt and pepper to taste

Instructions
1. Preheat the oven to 450 degrees F.
2. Pat the roasting chicken dry with paper towels. Season the inside with salt and pepper. Stuff the cavity of the chicken with the oregano and thyme bunches and with the pierced lemon.
3. Truss the chicken with kitchen twine on the ends of the drumsticks.
4. Massage half of the butter all over the chicken's skin. Season the chicken with salt and pepper. Do this on both sides.
5. Put the chicken on the pan with breast-side down.
6. Put in the oven and roast for 15 minutes at 450 degrees F. Then, turn the heat down to 325 degrees F and roast for 45 minutes.
7. Take the pan and chicken from the oven to flip the bird with its breasts facing up this time.
8. With a brush, baste the chicken with its own juices from the pan.
9. Sprinkle the chicken with the dried parsley and marjoram. Then, with a

patting motion, brush the chicken with it more of its juices.
10. Add the Brussel sprouts to the pan and toss it to coat it with the juices in it. Brush the tops of the Brussel sprouts and season with salt and pepper.
11. Put it back in the oven to roast for 40 minutes or until the chicken is browned and reaches an internal temperature of 165 degrees F.
12. Take it out of the oven and rest for 15 minutes. Serve.

Mississippi Roast

Cooking Time: 10 hours
Calories: 518
Servings: 8

Ingredients
- 3.8 lb beef chuck roast
- 16 oz deli-sliced pepperoncini
- 1 cup of brine from the pepperoncini
- ½ cup butter
- 2 tbsp powdered chicken bouillon
- 1 tbsp dried chives
- 1 tbsp dried parsley

- 1 tbsp onion powder
- 1 tbsp garlic powder
- 1 tbsp dried dill
- ½ tsp salt
- ¼ tsp freshly ground black pepper

Instructions
1. Put the roast in the slow cooker. Top the roast with the pepperoncini and pour the cup of the brine in the slow cooker.
2. Add the rest of the ingredients, except the butter, into the slow cooker and mix.
3. Put the butter on top of the roast.
4. Cover the slow cooker and cook it on high for 8 to 10 hours.
5. When the chuck roast looks like its falling apart, take it out of the slow cooker and shred it with two forks. The leftover juices can be stored and used for other recipes. Serve with mashed cauliflower or your favorite salad recipe.

Coconut-Lime Skirt Steak

Cooking Time: 20 minutes
Calories: 559
Servings: 5

Ingredients
- 2 lbs skirt steak
- ½ cup coconut oil, melted
- 2 tbsp freshly squeezed lime juice
- 1 tbsp minced garlic
- 1 tsp red pepper flakes
- 1 tsp grated fresh ginger
- ¾ tsp sea salt
- Zest from one lime

Instructions
1. In a large bowl, mix the coconut oil, lime zest and oil, ginger, garlic, red pepper flakes, and salt. This will be the marinade for the skirt steak.
2. Add the steak into the bowl and rub the marinade all over it. Let it marinate for at 20 minutes at room temperature. The coconut oil might harden but this is normal and expected.
3. Heat a large skillet over medium-high heat and sear the steak on both sides. Add the marinade into the skillet and cook it with the rest of the steak. Each side would take around 4 to 5 minutes to cook.

4. Slice according to your preference and serve.

Deconstructed Pizza Casserole

Cooking Time: 30 minutes
Calories: 504
Servings: 4

Ingredients
- 20 oz raw turkey Italian sausage, taken out of casings
- 15 oz tomatoes, sliced into medium-sized dices
- 10 oz fresh mushrooms, thickly sliced
- 15 slices of pepperoni
- 1 ½ cups grated mozzarella cheese
- 4 tsp olive oil
- ½ tsp dried oregano
- Salt and pepper to taste

Instructions
1. Preheat oven to 400 degrees F.
2. In a large frying pan, heat 2 tsp of the olive oil over medium-high heat. Cook the sausage until brown while making

sure that the ground meat is thoroughly cooked by breaking any chunks apart.
3. Coat a casserole dish sized 8x11 inches with olive oil.
4. Make a layer of the cooked sausage meat at the bottom of the casserole dish. On top of it, spread a layer of the diced tomatoes.
5. Season it with the oregano, salt, and pepper.
6. Wipe the pan of any remaining grease and heat it up over medium-high heat. Use the remaining olive oil to cook the mushrooms on it. Make sure to move around the mushrooms in the pan to make sure all sides are properly cooked and showing a brown color.
7. Create a layer of mushrooms on top of the tomato layer in the casserole. Sprinkle this layer with the grated mozzarella then evenly cover with the pepperoni slices.
8. Put it in the oven to cook for 25 minutes. You would want to get the

layer of cheese melted and a little bit browned.
9. Serve while hot.

Cabbage Lasagna

Cooking Time: 30 minutes
Calories: 639
Servings: 10

Ingredients
- 1 head of cabbage
- 3 lbs ricotta
- 2 lbs ground meat
- 40 oz unsweetened marinara sauce
- 32 oz shredded mozzarella
- 3 large eggs
- 1 ½ cups grated parmesan cheese
- ¼ cup grated parmesan cheese (separate)
- ¼ cup dried parsley

Instructions
1. Peel the leaves from the cabbage head. Make sure that the leaves stay intact and keep any tearing at a minimum or, if possible, none at all. Lightly boil the

leaves in salted water for 5 minutes. Drain and pat the leaves dry of any water.
2. Crack the eggs in a large mixing bowl and mix it with the ricotta, 1 ½ cups of grated parmesan, and parsley. Set aside.
3. In another bowl, stir the browned meat and marinara sauce together.
4. At the bottom of an 11x15 inch baking pan, spread ¾ cup of the meat and sauce mixture.
5. Place a layer of cabbage over the first layer of sauce.
6. Spread over the cabbage leaves about half of the ricotta cheese mixture you had set aside.
7. Top the ricotta cheese layer with another layer of the meat and sauce mixture.
8. Cover this layer of the meat and sauce mixture with half of the mozzarella.
9. Repeat the layers again from steps 4 to 7.

10. Top with the ¼ cup of parmesan cheese.
11. Put the pan in the oven and bake for around 25 minutes or until the cheese starts to brown.

Cheddar-Wrapped Taco Rolls

Cooking Time: 45 minutes
Calories: 511
Servings: 4

Ingredients

For the taco meat:

- 1 lb lean ground beef
- 2/3 cup water
- 1 ½ tbsp tomato paste
- 1 tbsp chili powder
- 1 pinch cayenne pepper
- ½ tsp cumin
- 1/3 tsp black pepper, freshly ground
- ¼ tsp salt
- ¼ tsp onion powder
- ¼ tsp paprika
- 1/8 tsp dried oregano
- 1/8 tsp garlic powder

For the taco seasoning:

- 2 tbsp chili powder
- ½ tsp freshly ground black pepper
- 2 tbsp cumin
- 2 tsp onion powder
- 2 tsp garlic powder
- 2 tsp celery salt
- ½ tsp cayenne pepper
- ½ tsp Himalayan Pink Salt

For the taco sauce:

- 8 oz Tomato Sauce
- ¼ cup water
- 3 tbsp taco seasoning
- 1 tbsp white vinegar
- 1 tbsp onion powder

For the taco:

- 1 cup taco meat
- 2 cups of cheddar cheese
- 1 cup taco meat, seasoned and cooked
- ½ cup avocado, chopped
- ¼ cup tomatoes, chopped
- 1 tsp taco sauce
- Optional toppings: onions and olives

Instructions

For the taco meat:
1. Heat a skillet to medium-high heat.
2. Brown the beef until there's barely no pink meat visible.
3. Mix in the rest of the ingredients.
4. Let it simmer for a few minutes in its own grease until it is no longer runny.

For the taco seasoning:
1. Combine all ingredients and mix well.
2. Store in an airtight spice jar.

For the taco sauce:
1. Heat a medium saucepan to medium heat.
2. Combine all ingredient in the saucepan.
3. Bring to a boil then reduce heat to low. Simmer for 5 to 10 minutes while stirring the contents of the saucepan occasionally.

For the taco:
1. Preheat oven to 400 degrees F.
2. Cover a baking sheet with lightly greased parchment paper. Sprinkle cheddar cheese on the parchment paper but make sure to leave space on the

edges so you can take out the cheese when done.
3. Put in the oven for 15 minutes or until the cheese bubbles and browns. Remove from the oven then remove the cheese from the parchment paper by lightly sliding a silicone spatula underneath edges then underneath the middle.
4. If spatula can't remove the cheese or is not solid enough, put it back in the oven until you can lift the cheese off the sheet.
5. Once you can lift the cheese from the sheet, add the taco meat and put it back in the oven for 5 to 10 minutes.
6. Combine the rest of the taco recipes in a bowl. Any other ingredients you add for toppings must be thin enough that you can wrap the taco in the end.
7. Remove the cheese and taco meet from the oven then add the toppings from the bowl in a thin layer on top of the meat and cheese.

8. Orient the longest edge of the sheet horizontally. With a pizza cutter, slice the cheese from top to bottom. Depending on the size of the sheet, this would usually give you 3-4 slices.
9. After making sure that the parchment paper isn't sticking to the cheese, roll each slice into taco rolls from bottom to top. Serve.

Lamb Meatballs with Cauliflower "Rice" Pilaf

Cooking Time: 25 minutes
Calories: 465
Servings: 4

Ingredients
- 200g cauliflower florets
- 4 oz. goat cheese, crumbled
- ½ yellow onion, chopped
- 4 cloves of garlic, minced
- 1 bunch of fresh mint leaves, roughly chopped
- 2 tbsp. coconut oil
- 1 tbsp. lemon zest

- Salt and Pepper to taste

For the meatballs:

- 1 lb ground lamb
- 1 large egg
- 1 tsp fennel seed
- 1 tsp paprika
- 1 tsp garlic powder
- 1 tsp salt
- 1 tsp pepper

Instructions

1. Put the cauliflower in a food processor and pulse it until it resembles rice. Cook it in a lightly oiled frying pan, cover, for about 8 minutes. Season with salt and pepper to taste.
2. In a large bowl, combine and thoroughly mix the lamb, egg, and spices for the meatballs. Form meatballs with the hands and set aside. This would yield around 12 to 15 meatballs.
3. Heat a skillet over medium heat. Grease with coconut oil and sauté the onion for 5 to 8 minutes or until it becomes translucent.

4. Add the garlic and cook until fragrant. Be careful not to burn the garlic.
5. Add the meatballs to the pan. Cook until all sides have no pinkish hue and firm to touch.
6. Divide cauliflower to 4 equal portions.
7. Divide the meatballs to the cauliflower rice portions. Top each portion with fresh mint leaves, lemon zest, and goat cheese. Serve.

Cheesy Spinach Rolls with Apple Slaw
Cooking Time: 20 minutes
Calories: 486
Servings: 4

Ingredients
For the crust:

- 2 ½ cups shredded low moisture mozzarella
- ½ cup Almond Flour
- 2 large eggs
- 6 tbsp Coconut flour

- ½ tsp salt

For the filling:

- 6 oz spinach leaves
- 4 oz cream cheese
- ¼ cup grated parmesan cheese
- 1 pinch salt

For the topping:

- ¾ cup coleslaw mix
- 1 apple, grated
- ¼ cup mayonnaise
- ¼ tsp salt

Instructions

1. Preheat the oven to 350 degrees F.
2. Using a large pan over medium-high heat and a bit of olive oil, wilt the spinach leaves.
3. Once the spinach leaves have wilted, add cream cheese and parmesan cheese then mix. Take it off the heat and set aside once the cheese have melted and mixed with the spinach leaves.

4. For the crust, soften the mozzarella in a bowl with the microwave. This would take at least 30 seconds.
5. Take out the bowl with mozzarella and add almond flour and coconut flour. Mix.
6. Add the eggs and salt. Thoroughly mix and combine the contents of the bowl until you get an even consistency.
7. Lay the crust mixture on a sheet of parchment paper and cover it with another sheet. Flatten the dough to an eighth of an inch with a rolling pin.
8. Cut the dough into 3x4 inch rectangles. Add ½ tsp of the filling on one side of each rectangle and roll or fold it over into a cigar shape.
9. Line a baking sheet with parchment paper and lightly grease it. Place the rolls on it with their seams down. Put it in the preheated oven for 15 minutes or until they become lightly golden brown.
10. Take the rolls out of the oven and let it cool for around 10 minutes.
11. In a bowl, mix the grated apple, coleslaw salad mix, mayonnaise, and

salt. Top it on the cooled cheesy spinach rolls. Serve.

Chicken and Bacon Patties

Cooking Time: 10 minutes
Calories: 655
Servings: 2

Ingredients

- 12 oz chicken breast, boiled
- 4 slices bacon, freshly fried to crisp
- 2 medium bell peppers, chopped
- 1 large egg
- ¼ cup sun-dried tomato pesto
- ¼ cup Parmesan
- 3 tbsp coconut flour

Instructions

1. In a food processor, put in the bell peppers until finely processed. Scoop out the mixture and, with paper towels, pat out excess moisture.
2. Put the chicken breast and bacon in the food processor and process until smooth.

3. Add the processed bell peppers, egg, parmesan, coconut floor, and tomato pesto into the food processor. Mix together the contents.
4. Take out the contents of the food processor and form patties with your hands.
5. Heat a frying pan over medium-high heat. Add some oil and fry the patties.
6. Once the bottom is browned, flip the patty and brown on the other side. Once cooked, remove from the pan and rest on paper towels.
7. Serve with salad.

Keto Quarter Pounder

Cooking Time: 10 minutes
Calories: 532
Servings: 2

Ingredients
- ½ pound ground beef
- 1 egg, beaten
- 1 strip bacon, roughly diced
- 2 cloves of garlic, peeled
- ½ tomato, roughly diced

- ¼ white onion, diced
- 2 slices of onion
- 2 slices of tomatoes
- 2 leaves of lettuce
- 2 tbsp butter
- 1 tbsp mayonnaise
- 1 tbsp sliced pickled jalapenos, roughly chopped
- 1 tbsp sriracha
- ½ tsp salt
- ½ tsp crushed red pepper
- ½ tsp basil
- ¼ tsp cayenne

Instructions

1. In a large mixing bowl, knead the ground beef with your hands for 3 minutes.
2. Finely grate the garlic onto the meat. Add in the egg, bacon, diced onion, jalapeno, tomato, mayonnaise, sriracha, salt, crushed red pepper, basil, and cayenne. Mix together and knead all the contents of the bowl for a few minutes.
3. Divide the mixture of meat into four equal parts and flatten each piece to

make 4 flat patties. Add a tablespoon of butter on the center of two patties and put the non-buttered patties on top of the buttered patties. Seal up the sides of the patties. This would leave you with only two patties in total.
4. On a pan or a grill, cook your patties and let the grease ooze out. DO NOT PRESS IT DOWN!
5. After 5 minutes, flip each patty and add the white onion slices on the pan or grill. On the two minute mark, flip the onions on their other side.
6. After 5 minutes, take out the patties and onions out of the pan. Lay out the lettuce leaves and place a patty on one half of each leaf.
7. Top each patty with a caramelized onion, a sliced tomato, sliced jalapenos, and mayonnaise. Fold the empty side of the lettuce over the patty and serve.

Pepperoni and Cheese on Cheese Crust Pizza
Cooking Time: 25 minutes

Calories: 400
Servings: 2

Ingredients

For the pizza crust:

- 1 ¼ cup shredded mozzarella cheese
- 1 egg
- 4 tbsp almond flour
- 3 tbsp coconut flour
- 1 tsp salt
- 1 tsp oregano
- 1 tsp crushed red pepper
- ½ tsp fennel seeds
- ½ tsp garlic powder

For the toppings:

- 6 oz mozzarella cheese, sliced
- ½ cup low-carb tomato basil pizza sauce
- 3 tbsp ricotta cheese
- 2 tbsp sliced jalapenos
- Pepperoni, your desired amount

Instructions

1. Preheat oven to 400 degrees F.
2. Melt the shredded mozzarella cheese in a microwave until soft.

3. Add almond flour, coconut flour, and egg. Mix all the ingredients together until it combines into a dough-like consistency.
4. Place the dough between two sheets of parchment paper and roll it into your desired pizza crust shape.
5. Discard the parchment paper on top and transfer to a baking sheet. Bake for at least 12 minutes. Take it out of the oven once it becomes slightly golden in color.
6. Evenly spread the sauce on the crust. Then, top it off with the cheese, ricotta, pepperoni, and jalapenos, respectively.
7. Put it back in the oven for at least 10 minutes. Take it out once the mozzarella has fully melted or until it gets a lightly golden color. Serve.

Cheddar Chicken and Broccoli Casserole

Cooking Time: 22 minutes
Calories: 529
Servings: 4

Ingredients
- 20 oz chicken breast, cooked
- 2 cups broccoli
- 1 cup cheddar cheese
- ½ cup sour cream
- ½ cup heavy cream
- 1 oz pork rinds, crushed
- 2 tbsp olive oil
- 1 tsp oregano
- ½ tsp paprika
- Salt and pepper to taste

Instructions
1. Preheat oven to 450 degrees F.
2. Blanche or steam the broccolis. Aim for a vibrant green color.
3. Shred the cooked chicken breasts into bite-sized pieces by pulling it apart with two forks.
4. In a large bowl, combine the shredded chicken breasts, broccoli, olive oil, and sour cream. Mix the contents well.
5. Lightly grease a baking dish that's big enough to spread the contents of the bowl in an even layer. Press the content firmly to the dish.

6. Top the layer of chicken mixture with cheddar cheese all the way to the edges of the baking dish.
7. Sprinkle the crushed pork rinds over the layer of shredded cheese.
8. Put the dish into the oven and bake for at least 20 minutes. When the casserole is bubbling slightly and gets browned on the edges, take it out and serve.

Ultimate Cheeseburger Loaf

Cooking Time: 45 minutes
Calories: 580
Servings: 4

Ingredients

For the beef filling:

- 12 oz ground beef
- 1 medium yellow onion, finely chopped
- 1 clove of garlic, crushed
- 2 tsp Worcestershire Sauce
- ½ tsp salt
- ¼ tsp pepper

For the dough:

- 1 ½ cups finely grated mozzarella cheese
- 1 ½ cups superfine almond flour
- 1 large egg
- ½ tsp xanthan gum
- 1 ½ tsp baking powder

For the filling:

- 14 slices of dill pickles
- ¼ red onion, sliced lengthwise
- 2 tbsp yellow mustard
- 1 ½ cup grated cheddar cheese

Instructions

For the beef filling:

Preheat oven to 375 degrees F.

1. Heat a large skillet to medium heat. Once the skillet is hot enough, put in the ground beef and break it up to smaller pieces with a fork. Stir the beef on the skillet until it is thoroughly browned.
2. Remove the beef from the skillet. Remove the grease except a tablespoon's worth of it from the skillet.

3. Put the skillet over medium heat and sauté the onions in it. Once the onions become soft and become brown on the edges, add the garlic. Continue sautéing for a minute then add the ground beef back into the skillet.
4. Stir in the Worcestershire sauce. Stir it and scrape the bottom of the skillet to render the flavor from it. Season with salt and pepper. Once the sauce has mostly evaporated, remove from heat. Taste and add seasoning if needed.

For the dough:

1. Set up a double boiler. With 2 inches of water in the lower part, turn the heat on high. Once it simmers, turn the heat to low.
2. In the top part, whisk almond flour, baking powder, and xanthan gum together. Stir in the egg and mozzarella cheese.
3. Frequently stir the mixture until the cheese melts and the mixture forms a dough-like ball. Be careful of the hot

surfaces and the steam from the bottom.
4. Transfer the dough on a sheet of parchment paper. Knead it to thoroughly incorporate almond flour into the dough and mix it with the cheese. Pat it into an oval shape. Cover with another sheet of parchment paper and roll it out to an oblong shape of about 12 by 15 inches in size. Straighten both parchments to prevent any wrinkles from forming in the dough.

For the loaf:

1. Spread lengthwise the ground beef filling on the middle third of the dough. Make sure to leave a third of the dough on both sides.
2. Drizzle mustard over the ground beef. Layer red onions and dill pickle slices over it. Top it all off with cheddar cheese.
3. Fold the two sides of the dough over the filling and seal the ends with your fingers. Crimp the seal similar to how

one would edge a pie. Pinch the ends and push down with a fork. With a sharp knife, pierce the dough along the sides of the seal for the steam to escape during baking.
4. Slide the parchment paper the dough is on onto a baking sheet. Put it in the preheated oven and bake for 25 to 30 minutes or until the loaf becomes golden brown. Let it cool for 5 minutes then transfer onto a cutting board and slice crosswise into 8 pieces. Serve hot.

Chapter 7
30 Whole Food Desserts Ketogenic Recipes

Coco Butter Fat Bombs

Prep Time: 20 minutes
Calories: 326
Servings: 2

Ingredients

- 4 tbsp extra-virgin coconut oil
- 4 tbsp cocoa powder
- 2 tbsp erythritol
- 4 tsp coconut butter, softened
- A pinch of Himalayan salt

Instructions

1. Mix together the cocoa powder, coconut oil, erythritol, and salt until no lumps are visible.

2. Evenly pour half of the cocoa mixture into 4 silicone cupcake molds. Put in the freezer for at least 5 minutes.
3. Spoon a teaspoon of coconut butter on top of each of the hardened cocoa mixture in the molds. Put back in the freezer for at least 5 minutes.
4. Cover the hardened coconut butter with the remaining cocoa mixture and put it back in the freezer for the last time for at least 5 minutes. Serve.

Berries and Cream Fat Bombs

Prep Time: 15 minutes
Calories: 336
Servings: 4

Ingredients
- 1 ½ cup coconut cream, canned or fresh
- 1 cup blueberries, preferably frozen
- 1 cup raspberries, preferably frozen
- 1 cup water
- 1 ½ tsp stevia
- ½ tsp vanilla extract

Instructions
1. In a small saucepan, boil the raspberries, half of the water, and ½ teaspoon of the stevia over medium high heat. Once it boils, reduce the heat to a medium low and simmer for 5 minutes.
2. Once the raspberries break down, remove from the heat and blend to a smooth puree with a blender or an immersion blender. Let it cool for later use.
3. Repeat the previous steps but this time with the blueberries.
4. In a small mixing bowl, mix the coconut cream, the vanilla extract, and half a teaspoon of the stevia.
5. Pour about 2 to 3 tablespoons of the raspberry puree into the popsicle molds. Put it in the freezer for at least an hour to set.
6. Next, pour about 3 to 4 tablespoons in of the coconut cream mixture in each mold, on top of the frozen raspberry

puree. Add the sticks and, again, freeze for at least an hour to set.
7. Lastly, add 2 to 3 tablespoons of blueberry puree in each mold. Put it back in the freezer for an hour or two. Once the popsicles are frozen and formed, serve.

Choco Peanut Butter Bombs

Prep Time: 10 minutes
Calories: 407
Servings: 4

Ingredients

- ½ cup extra virgin coconut oil
- ¼ cup shredded coconut
- ¼ cup cocoa powder
- 6 tbsp hemp seeds
- 4 tbsp peanut butter powder
- 2 tbsp heavy cream
- 28 drops liquid stevia
- 1 tsp. vanilla extract

Instructions

1. Mix into a paste the coconut oil and all of the dry ingredients.

2. Add the heavy cream, liquid stevia, and vanilla extract into the coconut oil paste mixture. Mix everything until ingredients are thoroughly combined and have a creamy consistency.
3. Roll the now creamy coconut paste into balls with your hands and coat it with the shredded coconuts.
4. On a tray lined with parchment paper, lay the rolled coconut paste and put in the freezer for around 20 minutes. When the balls become hard enough to retain its shape, the choco peanut butter bombs are ready to serve.

No-Bake Choco Peanut Butter Fudge
Prep Time: 10 minutes
Calories: 379
Servings: 6

Ingredients
- ¾ cup unsweetened peanut butter
- 1/3 cup unsalted grass-fed butter
- 100g baking dark chocolate
- 2 tbsp erythritol
- 1 tsp vanilla extract

Instructions

1. In a saucepan, melt the chocolate and the butter.
2. Stir into the saucepan the peanut butter and the erythritol.
3. Line a small container with parchment paper and pour the contents of the pan into it.
4. Put the container in the freezer for at least 30 minutes or until the mixture sets.
5. Once it sets, cut it into desired size. Serve or store in the freezer.

Chai Spice Mug Cake

Prep Time: 1 minute
Calories: 297
Servings: 1

Ingredients

For the base:
- 1 large egg
- 2 tbsp almond flour
- 2 tbsp grass-fed unsalted butter
- 1 tbsp erythritol
- ½ tsp baking powder

- 7 drops liquid stevia

For the flavor:

- 2 tbsp almond flour
- ¼ tsp ginger powder
- ¼ tsp ground cinnamon
- ¼ tsp ground clove
- ¼ tsp ground cardamom pods
- ¼ tsp vanilla extract

Instructions

1. Combine all the base ingredients in a mug. Mix until all ingredients are thoroughly combined.
2. Add the flavor ingredients in the mug. Mix until combined.
3. Put it in the microwave and set it on high for around 70 seconds.
4. Turn mug upside on a plate and tap the bottom to take the finished cake out of it. Top with sugar-free whipped cream and cinnamon powder.

Mug Churro
Prep Time: 1 minute

Calories: 298
Servings: 1

Ingredients

For the base:

- 1 large egg
- 2 tbsp almond flour
- 2 tbsp grass-fed unsalted butter
- 1 tbsp erythritol
- ½ tsp baking powder
- 7 drops liquid stevia

For the flavor:

- 2 tbsp almond flour
- ¼ tsp ground nutmeg
- ¼ tsp ground cinnamon
- ¼ tsp vanilla extract
- 1/8 tsp all spice powder
- 1/8 tsp ginger powder

Instructions

1. Combine all the base ingredients in a mug. Mix until all ingredients are thoroughly combined.
2. Add the flavor ingredients in the mug. Mix until combined.

3. Put it in the microwave and set it on high for around 70 seconds.
4. Turn mug upside on a plate and tap the bottom to take the finished cake out of it. Top with sugar-free whipped cream and cinnamon powder.

PB Choco Chunk in a Mug
Prep Time: 1 minute
Calories: 387
Servings: 1

Ingredients
For the base:

- 1 large egg
- 2 tbsp almond flour
- 2 tbsp grass-fed unsalted butter
- 1 tbsp erythritol
- ½ tsp baking powder
- 7 drops liquid stevia

For the flavor:

- 10g baker's dark chocolate
- 1 tbsp unsweetened peanut butter
- ½ tsp vanilla extract

Instructions

1. Combine all the base ingredients in a mug. Mix until all ingredients are thoroughly combined.
2. Add the flavor ingredients in the mug. Mix until combined.
3. Put it in the microwave and set it on high for around 70 seconds.
4. Turn mug upside on a plate and tap the bottom to take the finished cake out of it. Top with sugar-free whipped cream.

Coco Choco Mocha Mug Cake

Prep Time: 1 minute
Calories: 300
Servings: 1

Ingredients

For the base:

- 1 large egg
- 2 tbsp almond flour
- 2 tbsp grass-fed unsalted butter
- 1 tbsp erythritol
- ½ tsp baking powder
- 7 drops liquid stevia

For the flavor:

- 1 tbsp coconut milk
- 1 tbsp cocoa powder
- 1 tbsp shredded coconut
- 2 tsp coconut flour
- ½ tsp fine fresh coffee grounds

Instructions
1. Combine all the base ingredients in a mug. Mix until all ingredients are thoroughly combined.
2. Add the flavor ingredients in the mug. Mix until combined.
3. Put it in the microwave and set it on high for around 70 seconds.
4. Turn mug upside on a plate and tap the bottom to take the finished cake out of it. Top with additional shredded coconut.

Pecan Butter Ice Cream
Prep Time: 25 minutes
Calories: 268
Servings: 6

Ingredients
- 1 ½ cup coconut milk, unsweetened
- ¼ cup crushed pecans
- ¼ cup heavy whipping cream
- 5 tbsp grass-fed butter
- 25 drops stevia
- ¼ tsp xanthan gum

Instructions
1. In a pan over low heat, melt the butter until it turns to an amber color.
2. Add heavy whipping cream, pecans, and stevia into the pan and stir to combine together.
3. Whisk the coconut milk and xanthan gum into the pan.
4. Pour in the mixture into an ice cream maker.
5. Follow the instructions on the manual of your ice cream maker.
6. Serve or store in the freezer in an airtight container.

Keto Strawberry Ice Cream
Prep Time: 25 minutes

Calories: 270
Servings: 3

Ingredients
- 1 cup strawberries, pureed
- 1 cup heavy whipping cream
- 3 large egg yolks
- 1/3 cup erythritol
- 1/2 tsp vanilla extract
- 1/8 tsp xanthan gum

Instructions
1. In a pot over low heat, dissolve the erythritol in the heavy cream.
2. In a large bowl, beat the egg yolks with an electric mixer until it doubles in amount. Add a few tablespoons of the heavy cream mixture to prevent the egg yolks from scrambling.
3. Once the egg mixture becomes warm, start to slowly add the heavy cream mixture while constantly beating the contents of the bowl.
4. Pour the contents of the bowl into an ice cream maker. Follow its instructions.

5. When the ice cream mixture is adequately chilled, mix in the blended strawberries. Chill in the freezer overnight. Serve.

Classic Vanilla Ice Cream

Prep Time: 25 minutes
Calories: 241
Servings: 2

Ingredients

- 2 ½ cups whipping cream
- ½ cup unsweetened almond milk
- ½ cup erythritol
- 1 tbsp vanilla extract

Instructions

1. In a large bowl, use an electric mixer to blend the whipping cream until it forms stiff peaks.
2. Add the erythritol and vanilla extract and whip the ingredients together until combined.
3. Add in the almond milk and blend the contents of the bowl until the mixture thickens.

4. Transfer contents to an ice cream maker and proceed according to its instructions.
5. Serve. Top with nuts or fruits if desired.

Mocha Pudding Cake

Cooking Time: 3 hours
Calories: 240
Servings: 8

Ingredients

- 5 large eggs
- ¾ cup grass-fed unsalted butter, cut to large chunks
- 2/3 cup erythritol
- 1/3 cup almond flour
- ½ cup heavy cream
- 2 oz unsweetened chocolate, finely chopped
- 4 tbsp unsweetened cocoa powder
- 2 tbsp fine fresh coffee grounds
- 1 tsp vanilla extract
- 1/8 tsp sea salt

Instructions

1. Grease the pot of the slow cooker with coconut oil.
2. In a small saucepan over low heat, melt the chocolate and the butter while occasionally whisking. Remove from heat to let it cool.
3. In a small bowl, whisk the cream, coffee grounds, and vanilla extract.
4. In another small bowl, mix together the cocoa powder, almond flour, and salt.
5. In a large bowl, beat the eggs with an electric mixer on high speed while gradually adding the erythritol until it gets a slightly thicker consistency. This would take about 5 minutes.
6. With the mixer on low, add the melted butter and chocolate mixture.
7. Then, add in the almond flour mixture.
8. Switch the mixer to medium speed and add the heavy cream mixture.
9. Pour the batter into the slow cooker and place a paper towel over the opening before covering it with the lid.

10. Cook on low for around 2 to 3 hours or until the center of the cake has a soft soufflé-like consistency. Serve with any of the previous ice cream recipes.

Keto Coffee Cake

Cooking Time: 3 hours
Calories: 240
Servings: 8

Ingredients

For the base:

- ¼ cup unflavored protein powder
- ¼ cup erythritol
- 6 large eggs
- 6 oz cream cheese
- 2 tsp vanilla extract
- ¼ tsp liquid stevia
- ¼ tsp cream of tartar

For the filling:

- 1 ½ cup almond flour
- ¼ cup butter
- 2 tsp maple syrup

- 2 ¼ tsp coconut oil
- ¾ cup water
- ½ tsp vanilla extract
- ¼ cup erythritrol
- ¼ cup butter
- 1 tbsp ground cinnamon

Instructions
1. Preheat the oven to 325 degrees F.
2. Separate the eggs yolks from the egg whites.
3. Cream the egg yolks with the erythritrol and the liquid stevia.
4. Add the cream cheese and the protein powder to the creamed yolks. Mix it together until the batter thickens.
5. Beat the egg whites with the cream of tartar until you get to form stiff peaks.
6. Fold together half of the egg whites mixture with half of the egg yolk mixture. Then fold the remaining egg white mixture and, then, the remaining egg yolk mixture into the combination.
7. Pour batter into a lightly sprayed round cake pan.

8. Mix all of the filling ingredients together until you get it to form a dough.
9. Take half of the filling dough and rip it to pieces. Push these pieces onto top the batter in the pan.
10. Put it into the oven to bake for 20 minutes.
11. After the 20 minutes, top the cake with the remainder of the filling.
12. Put it back into the oven for an additional 20-30 minutes. Check for doneness with a toothpick. If it comes out clean, it's done.
13. Remove from the oven and let cool for at least 20 minutes before removing from the pan.

Chapter 8

Snack Ketogenic Recipes

Spicy Cheese and Sausage Dip

Cooking Time: 2 hours
Calories: 191
Servings: 20

Ingredients
- 1 lb hot Italian ground sausage
- 16 oz sour cream
- 8 oz pepper jack cheese, diced
- 8 oz cream cheese
- 1 ¾ cup diced tomatoes
- ¼ cup diced habaneros
- ¼ cup white onions

Instructions
1. Cook the sausage in a saucepan over medium heat.
2. Once it becomes lightly browned, add the onions in the saucepan. T
3. Take the saucepan off the stovetop once the sausage is fully browned.
4. Layer the cream cheese and the pepper jack cheese at the bottom of a slow cooker's stoneware.
5. Pour the sausage and onion on top of the cheese layer.
6. Pour and spread on top of the sausage and onion the sour cream.
7. Set the slow cooker on high and let it cook for about an hour then thoroughly mix the contents of the stoneware.
8. Continue cooking in the slow cooker for a total of two hours.
9. Serve it with your favorite vegetable or no-carb bread sticks and carb-free chips or crackers.

Cheesy Onion Dip
Cooking Time: 15 minutes

Calories: 125
Servings: 10

Ingredients

- 1 lb cauliflower, whole
- 1 ½ cup chicken broth
- ¾ cup cream cheese, cut into chunks
- ½ cup diced onion
- ¼ cup sugar-free mayonnaise
- ½ tsp garlic powder
- ½ tsp chili powder
- ½ tsp ground cumin
- ½ tsp freshly ground black pepper
- ½ tsp sea salt

Instructions

1. Simmer until tender the cauliflower and onion in the chicken broth. Stir in the ground or powdered spices.
2. Once the cauliflower and onion are soft and tender, whisk in the cream cheese until it melts.
3. Blend the mixture with a stick blender or in the blender until it gets a smooth consistency.

4. Thoroughly whisk mayonnaise into the mixture.
5. Chill in the refrigerator for 2 to 3 hours before serving.

Pizza Dip

Cooking Time: 15 minutes
Calories: 225
Servings: 4

Ingredients
- 4 oz cream cheese
- 1 cup shredded mozzarella cheese
- ½ cup tomato sauce
- ¼ cup sugar-free mayonnaise
- ¼ cup sour cream
- ¼ cup parmesan
- Salt and pepper to taste

Instructions
1. Preheat oven to 350 degrees F.
2. Microwave the cream cheese until it reaches room temperature.
3. In a mixing bowl, mix together the sour cream, mozzarella cheese, and mayonnaise into the cream cheese.

4. Divide the mixture between 4 small baking-proof ceramic bowls (also known as ramekins) and drop 2 tbsp. worth of tomato sauce on top of each.
5. Divide the mozzarella and parmesan between the ramekins. Evenly sprinkle on top of the sauce.
6. Bake for at least 15 minutes or until the dip is bubbling.
7. Let it cool and serve with your vegetable sticks or keto breadsticks.

"Bread" Sticks

Cooking Time: 15 minutes
Calories: 215
Servings: 6

Ingredients

For the dough:

- 2 cups shredded mozzarella cheese
- ¾ cup almond flour
- 1 large egg
- 3 tbsp cream cheese
- 1 tbsp psyllium husk powder
- 1 tsp baking powder

For the flavoring:

- 2 tbsp Italian seasoning
- 1 tsp salt
- 1 tsp freshly ground pepper

Instructions
1. Preheat oven to 400 degrees F.
2. Combine egg and cream cheese in a bowl.
3. In a separate bowl, combine the dry ingredients.
4. Microwave mozzarella cheese until sizzling.
5. Mix together all the ingredients in a large mixing bowl until it forms a dough-like consistency.
6. Knead the dough with your hands to thoroughly combine the ingredients together.
7. Cut it into shapes and season with the flavoring.
8. Put it in the oven to bake for 15 minutes or until dough becomes crisp.
9. Serve the breadstick warm with your favorite dip.

Kale Chips

Cooking Time: 12 minutes
Calories: 207
Servings: 1

Ingredients

- 1 large bunch of kale, washed and patted dry
- 2 tbsp coconut or olive oil
- 1 tbsp sea salt

Instructions

1. Preheat oven to 350 degrees F.
2. Remove the kale from its stems.
3. In a Ziploc bag, shake very well the kale with the oil.
4. Lay and spread out the kale on a baking sheet. Flatten each leaf on the baking sheet.
5. Cook it in the oven for 12 minutes then season with salt. Serve.

Green Bean Fries

Cooking Time: 10 minutes
Calories: 375

Servings: 1

Ingredients

- 12 oz green beans, snipped and patted dry
- 2/3 cup grated parmesan
- 1 large egg
- ½ tsp Himalayan salt
- ½ tsp garlic powder
- ¼ tsp black pepper
- ¼ tsp paprika

Instructions

1. Preheat oven to 400 degrees F.
2. In a shallow plate, evenly mix the parmesan, salt, garlic powder, paprika, and black pepper.
3. In a bowl, whisk the egg.
4. Drench the green beans in the egg and let the excess drip off.
5. Then, press the drenched green beans in the parmesan mixture. Evenly coat all sides of the green beans.
6. Lay the green beans on a baking sheet. Make sure to avoid overcrowding and

that the green beans have space between each other.
7. Bake in the oven for around 10 minutes or until slightly golden.
8. Serve with your favorite dressing or dip.

Tropical Smoothie

Prep Time: 2 minutes
Calories: 189
Servings: 4

Ingredients

- ¾ cup unsweetened coconut milk
- ¼ cup sour cream
- 7 large ice cubes
- 2 tbsp golden flaxseed meal
- 1 tbsp MCT or coconut oil
- ¼ tsp mango extract
- ¼ tsp banana extract
- ¼ tsp blueberry extract
- 20 drops stevia

Instructions

1. Put all the ingredients in the blender.
2. Let it sit for the flax meal to soak up some moisture.

3. Blend for two minutes. Serve.

Spinach and Cucumber Smoothie

Prep Time: 2 minutes
Calories: 215
Servings: 2

Ingredients

- 2.5 oz cucumber, peeled and cubed
- 1 cup unsweetened coconut milk
- 2 handfuls of spinach
- 7 large ice cubes
- 1 tbsp MCT or coconut oil
- ¼ tsp xanthan gum
- 12 drops stevia

Instructions

1. Put all the ingredients in a blender and blend for 2 minutes.
2. Serve.

Hearty Red Smoothie

Prep Time: 2 minutes
Calories: 190
Servings: 1

Ingredients

- 1 cup chopped red cabbage
- ½ cup raspberries
- 8 oz cold water
- 5 medium strawberries
- 1 roma tomato
- 1 large ice cube
- ½ red bell pepper

Instructions

1. Put all the ingredients in a blender and blend for 2 minutes.
2. Serve.

Green Smoothie

Prep Time: 2 minutes
Calories: 193
Servings: 2

Ingredients

- 3 cups water
- 2 cups spinach, frozen or fresh
- 2 tbsp chia seeds
- 2 tbsp golden flax seed meal
- 1 tbsp MCT or coconut oil
- 7 large ice cubes

Instructions
1. Put all the ingredients in a blender and blend for 2 minutes.
2. Serve.

Conclusion

With these recipes, you can follow the ketogenic diet without sacrificing good food. There may be times in which you'll fail to maintain it but as long as you get back to it, you will eventually achieve and maintain the shape you desire.

The ketogenic diet is originally meant for people with certain ailments and, therefore, has its risks involved. If the diet is affecting your healthy in any negative or unusual way, it is better to seek advice and guidance from your doctor. Your wellbeing is always the priority and it is more important than any diet that you're following.

In closing, I wish you the best of luck in your pursuit of health and in all your endeavors.

Printed in Great Britain
by Amazon